Lectins – A 360° Analys

Why Lectins make you sick ar
our Lectin intake to live more healthy lives –
background, guidelines, dietary change, recipes

©2019, Lutz Schneider

Published by Expertengruppe Verlag

The contents of this book have been written with great care. However, we cannot guarantee the accuracy, comprehensiveness and topicality of the subject matter. The contents of the book represent the personal experiences and opinions of the author. No legal responsibility or liability will be accepted for damages caused by counter-productive practices or errors of the reader. There is also no guarantee of success. The author, therefore, does not accept responsibility for lack of success, using the methods described in this book.

All information contained herein is purely for information purposes. It does not represent a recommendation or application of the methods mentioned within. This book does not purport to be complete, nor can the topicality and accuracy of the book be guaranteed. This book in no way replaces the competent recommendations of, or care given by a doctor. The author and publisher do not take responsibility for inconvenience or damages caused by use of the information contained herein.

Lectins – A 360° Analysis

Why Lectins make you sick and how we can reduce our Lectin intake to live more healthy lives – background, guidelines, dietary change, recipes

Published by Expertengruppe Verlag

TABLE OF CONTENTS

About the author 11

Preface 13

What are Lectins? 20

    Introduction to Lectins 20

    Lectins and blood groups 22

    Different types of Lectins 23

        Legumes: 24

        Grain: 24

        Nightshade (Solanaceae) plants: 25

        Fungi/Mushroom: 25

        Bulbous plants 26

        Fruits 26

        Lectin in grain 27

    What happens in our intestines? 30

What happens outside our intestines? 32

Lectins causing disorders and diseases 33

Positive characteristics of Lectins 36

The Leaky Gut Syndrome 37

How are the bowels structured? 38

What is the leaky gut syndrome? 41

How do you recognise leaky gut syndrome? 44

Which autoimmune diseases does it cause? 45

How is it diagnosed? 46

   Who can diagnose a leaky gut syndrome? 47

   What is tested? 48

   Who treats the leaky gut syndrome? 53

What should you be aware of with leaky gut syndrome? 55

   Lectins 56

   Sugar 58

   Fast Food 59

- Alcohol 60
- Sport 61
- Stress 62
- Food allergens 63
- Medications 64

Diet for leaky gut syndrome 65
- Food supplements and nutrients for leaky gut syndrome. 66

Diet without Lectins 68
- The Gundry Theory 68
  - About Steven R. Gundry 69
  - Success in the treatment of diseases 70
- List of foods 72
  - Positive foods 73
  - Negative foods 82
- Casein A2 Milk 86

What is the difference between A1 and A2 milk? 87

What happens during digestion of A1 milk?..... 88

Why is there a difference between A1 and A2 milk? 89

Why is this not well-known?............................. 90

Where do I find A2 milk products? 91

Making Lectins harmless 92

Cooking for long enough 93

Peeling and core removal 94

Steeping 95

Fermenting.. 98

Cooking in the pressure cooker 102

Further tips for every day 103

Avoid high-Lectin foods................................... 103

Enjoy high-Lectin foods sparingly 104

- This is how you optimise the health benefits of potatoes. 106
- Safe Lectins 107
- White grain instead of brown 108

Changing your diet, step by step 109
- Phase 1: Cleansing/restoration 110
  - Food plan for 3 days:.. 111
- Phase 2: Repair and restore 118
  - Rules during Phase 2: 120
- Phase 3: Reap the rewards 122
  - Intermittent fasting.. 124
- The Keto Intensive Care Programme 126
- Other disruptive factors which disable a healthy gut 127
  - Broad spectrum antibiotics.............................. 128
  - Non-steroidal anti-inflammatory drugs (NSAIDs) 129

Gastric acid blocking agents (Proton pump inhibitors, PPI) 130

Artificial sweeteners 131

Hormone system Disruptors 132

Genetic modified Organisms (GMO): 134

Blue light: 135

Losing weight without Lectins 136

Why low-carb diets do not help long-term 137

The paleo concept 138

The Keto diet 140

Recipes 141

Breakfast 141

Crunchy muesli 141

Sunday bread buns 143

Smoothies 145

Green Smoothie 145

Avocado Fig Smoothie 147

Snacks 148

   Cabbage Crisps 148

   Coconut yoghurt with dried fruit 150

   Romaine lettuce boats filled with guacamole 152

Main courses 153

   Asia Wrap with chicken and coriander dip 153

   Roasted broccoli with cauliflower rice and sautéed onions 156

   Cabbage kale sautée with salmon and avocado 159

   Lentil salad with sesame dressing 161

   Romaine salad with avocado and basil pesto chicken 164

   Rocket salad with chicken and lemon vinaigrette 167

   Lemony Brussel sprouts, kale and onions with cabbage steak 169

Conclusion 171

Did you enjoy my book? 176

References..178

Book Recommendations 180

Disclaimer..186

ABOUT THE AUTHOR

Lutz Schneider lives with his wife, Doris, in an old farmhouse in beautiful Rhineland.

Ever since he studied the biology of evolution, over 20 years ago, he has been interested in marginal health subjects, which are often hidden from the main stream, but which are scientifically well accepted. He teaches this knowledge, not only to his students, but also reaches a wider audience in Germany with his various publications.

In his books, he speaks about subjects, the positive effects of which are widely unknown and on which he can pass on his own experiences. All of his publications, therefore, are based on indisputable scientific facts, but also encompass his own very personal experiences and knowledge. This way, the reader not only receives factual information about the subject but also a practical guide with a wide range of knowledge and useful tips, which are easy to understand and put into practice.

Lutz Schneider's easy to read work puts the reader into a relaxed and pleasant ambience, while gaining insight into a subject which few know anything about but which everyone could profit from.

PREFACE

Intolerances, such as Lactose, Gluten, Sorbitol, Histamines or Fructose are well-known. But have you ever heard of Lectins? If not, you are probably thinking *here comes the next diet trend*. In reality, it is a form of nutrition which is slowly becoming better known. Lectins are substances which are not well absorbed into the body and which can cause discomfort or sickness. Lectins do not belong to the classical group of intolerances. However, if you eat low-lectin foods, a whole range of intolerances can be reduced, all at once.

Glutens belong, for example, to the Lectin group. Cows, which are commonly used for milk products in Europe, carry a gene mutation which makes the milk rich in lectins, and also sugar, which is responsible for Fructose intolerance, contains Lectins.

These days, many of us suffer from intolerances and abdominal discomfort. But why is it happening so frequently? Are we wrong in our assumptions on nutritional theories about what is healthy and unhealthy for our stomachs? In this book, we will answer many such questions and will examine what lies behind Lectins. Why are these substances found in plants and what do they do to humans? We have probably underestimated these small substances or not yet completely understood them.

It is a complex subject but it makes sense if you look at the detail. I will explain what Lectins do to our bowels and how that connects to autoimmune disease and other such disorders.

This subject is very important to me, because I also suffered a long time from abdominal pain. I know what it means to have digestion problems and the doctors do not know what is causing them. Over the years, I have tried many types of diets and I kept a symptom log book about my nutrition. For a long time, I went without Glutens, Sorbitol, Fructose, Lactose and Histamines, each in isolation. That meant that I had gone without each of these substances, separately, for a while and observed my reaction. I noticed some improvement in my symptoms, particularly with Gluten, but the problem was not completely solved. I continued to have abdominal pain, flatulence and diarrhoea. In addition, I often felt tired and washed-out.

I visited many different doctors of traditional medicine during this time. I often heard that the symptoms were triggered psychologically, or the diagnosis was IBS (irritable bowel syndrome) or something similar. I failed to find a solution or a suitable diet.

It was only after consultation with a holistic health practitioner, that I thought of a different idea. He explained to me about "leaky gut syndrome". Often, this is connected to food intolerances, such as Lectins, and can cause disorders. This was the first time I had heard about Lectins. Before this, I had not heard anything about them.

The information which I received matched my symptoms and could explain why a diet, which only addressed one category of intolerance, did not improve my condition.

Firstly, I wanted to know more about the subject. I noticed quickly that it is a large and interesting topic and that American pioneer, Steven Gundry, was the first to recognise that there was a connection between heart diseases, autoimmune diseases and Lectin.

If you are seeking information about Lectins, you are bound to bump into the name Gundry and his work. My literature is partly based on the findings of Gundry and his nutrition theory.

Today, there are so many diseases which are directly connected to nutrition. However, the basic diets of today do not come under as much scrutiny as they perhaps should. Surprisingly, wheat is not good for our bowels and particularly wholemeal products which are even worse than white flour products. I will explain why this is the case later in the book. I was also told that vegetables, which are thought to be healthy, are not always what they seem. Here, there was a danger of which I was previously not aware.

I have changed my eating habits according to Gundry and continue to base my diet upon it. I would like to pass my practical experience on to you. It is not to be perceived as a diet, but as a form of nutrition which should become part of your everyday life.

If you are looking for a change in eating habits which will help you to gain control over your abdominal problems and live a symptom-free life, I can show you what you need to do, based on my own experiences. You will notice quickly how well the advice can be adapted into everyday life. It is not witchcraft. You have already taken the first step by acquiring information about the subject. That knowledge and the understanding of it are the foundation for your new eating plan.

This book offers you a comprehensive list of foods which have positive and negative effects and which contain more Lectin and which contain less. You will also find tips on which specific foods are recommended in different phases of your diet change. In Phase 1, fewer foods are permitted but that number will increase significantly in Phase 2. The literature originates from Gundry, which has been supplemented a later work, originally in German, by Konstantin Kirsch. You can find a reference to the source in the appendix. The completeness and accuracy of the information contained therein is free of liability. I have personally been following these dietary recommendations for some time and have found them to be very helpful. This is why I decided to adopt them for this book. The list of foods written by Gundry is much more detailed than similar dietary options written by other people. This is useful when changing your eating habits, particularly at the beginning, when you are trying to find your way. Later, you will not rely on the list very much as you will have internalised the positive and negative foods.

In the recipes, you will always find a note as to which phase the foods are recommended for. This makes it easier to start off and to get an idea what you can do with the foods which you are permitted to eat. In the first phase, it seems that there is a lot of cabbage or other things which may seem daunting. I promise you that the recipes taste better than they sound. I personally found a new love of cabbage during my dietary change. I hope I can also interest you in newly or rediscovered tastes and show you how versatile and tasty the recipes can be.

Perhaps you experienced, as I did, that a doctor was also not able to give you the right type of advice. I hope that my book can give you a new insight into what is happening inside your body and how it reacts to certain substances. I hope I can also show you an alternative path to enhance and support your health by optimising your nutrition.

With this book, I would like to draw your attention to how we can influence our own health through our nutrition. We can protect our bowels against damage and other diseases by eating the correct foods. In this way we can positively influence diseases and be less dependent upon medicinal therapies.

I hope you enjoy reading my book and wish you success in your dietary change. Remember that a new dietary option is always a challenge, because you must leave your old habits behind and start on a new path. Allow yourself some time until you have got used to the new recipes and tastes. I am sure that this type of nutrition will help you to restore balance to your bowels and improve your health in the long term.

WHAT ARE LECTINS?

INTRODUCTION TO LECTINS

Lectins are glycoproteins. They belong to the group of secondary plant compounds and are known as the "anti-nutrients".

Anti-nutrients are – as the name suggests – the opposite of nutrients. Instead of being good for humans and animals, they negatively impact organisms. These anti-nutrient components are secondary plant compounds, which can be found in grain and legumes.

Lectins are mostly to be found in plants but can also be found in animal products. The main issue is that plants have the ability to protect themselves. This prevents them from being eaten by animals or humans. Animals and insects which eat those foods can develop diseases which they could die from. Consequently, animals should avoid these plants. You could call it a passive defence to ensure survival.

In addition, Lectins protect plants from micro-organisms which are damaging to them, such as fungi, certain diseases and pests.

The concentration of Lectins is particularly high in the seeds. You can also find them to a lesser extent in other plant tissue, such as tubers, bulbs, rootstocks and bark. They have both harmful and beneficial characteristics for humans.

LECTINS AND BLOOD GROUPS

In the 1940s, William Boyd determined that the protein Agglutinin in lima beans agglutinates (clumps) the red corpuscles in human blood group A, but not in blood groups 0 or B. In reality, he had discovered that these Agglutinins specifically effected particular blood groups. Together with Elizabeth Shapely he became responsible for the term "Lectins", which comes from the Latin word meaning "select" or "choose".

In medicine today, Lectins are used to determine blood groups because they can bind with carbohydrates and glycoproteins. This ability is useful for the development of medicines, which are meant to be absorbed into particular cells.

DIFFERENT TYPES OF LECTINS

"Lectin" is a general term for various types of sugar-protein compounds. Every type of plant has a different Lectin. However, their characteristics and impact are similar, so that they can be referred to, collectively, as Lectins. In the following summary, you will find examples of various Lectins. Of all the Lectins, the most researched are the PHA (Phyto-haemagglutinins) and WGA (Wheat Germ Agglutinins).

LEGUMES:

Lectin	Food
Phytohaemagglutinin (PHA)	Red kidney beans
Soybean agglutinin (SBA) und Soybean lectin (SBL)	Soybeans
Broad bean agglutinin, Vicia faba agglutinin (VFA)	Broad beans
Phaseolus vulgaris leucoagglutinin	Green beans
Concanavalin A (ConA)	Jack beans
Cicer arietinum agglutinin (CAA-I und CAA-II)	Chick peas
Lens culinaris lectin (LCL)	Lentils
Pisum sativum agglutinin (PSA)	Peas
Peanut lectin (PNA)	Peanuts

GRAIN:

Lectin	Food

Wheat germ agglutinin (WGA)	Wheat (Wheat germ)
Rice bran agglutinin (RBA)	Rice (Rice bran)
Corn coleoptile lectin (CLL)	Corn

NIGHTSHADE (SOLANACEAE) PLANTS:

Lectin	**Food**
Solanum tuberosum lectin (STL)	Potatoes
Lycopersicon esculentum lectin (LEL, TL)	Tomatoes

FUNGI/MUSHROOM:

Lectin	**Food**
Pleurotus ostreatus lectin (POL)	Oyster mushrooms
Agaricus bisporus agglutinin (ABA)	White mushrooms

BULBOUS PLANTS

Lectin	Food
Allium sativum lectin (ASA I und ASA II)	Garlics
Allium cepa agglutinin (ACA)	Onions

FRUITS

Lectin	Food
Banana lectin (BanLec-I)	Bananas

LECTIN IN GRAIN

There is a Lectin called Wheat Germ Agglutinin or WGA, present in wheat, which is particularly treacherous. Its molecules attach themselves to the body's own protein molecules so that the body's molecules appear hostile; or the attacking molecules hide behind the body's own molecules (mimicry). When the immune system produces antibodies to fight the "enemy", the antibodies also attach themselves to the body's own molecules: An auto-immune reaction occurs as the immune system attacks the body's own protein. It can randomly attack one specific body's protein, which makes the auto-immune disease so diverse (and therefore difficult to research).

There is, for example, detailed research on this process and its connection to rheumatoid arthritis and the autoimmune variant of arthritis. A similar connection has been made for autoimmune diseases of the thyroid glands.

The list of autoimmune diseases connected to grain is getting longer because the type of cell affecting Lectins is random. The type of damage which is caused by an individual's immune system is equally random.

A good example of this can be found in the animal world. Elephants, living in the wild, only feed from the leaves of the trees in their own environment. As far as we know, African elephants do not suffer from coronary vascular diseases. However, where their wooded environment is being destroyed, many elephants are being fed with hay and grain. Among these animals, 50 percent suffer from severe damage to their coronary artery. This is said to be caused by the Lectins in the grain, which never should have been in their diet and which adhere to their arteries, causing heart attacks.

With this example I would like to show you which sugar molecule of the Lectin WGA (wheat germ agglutinin) is involved. It has been discovered that humans, just like elephants, have a specific molecule which causes the problem. These molecules are called Neu5Ac and they attach themselves to the inside wall of the artery, just as enterocytes, which are responsible for resorption of the nutrients into the body, attach themselves to the intestinal wall. Most other mammals have a different kind of sugar molecule, called Neu5Gc. A gene mutation, which happened during the separation of humans from other primates about 8 million years ago, caused humans (and elephants) to lose their ability to synthesize Neu5Gc. Chimpanzees, however, have retained this ability.

Lectins, particularly those from grain, attach themselves to Neu5Ac but cannot attach to Neu5Gc. This is why chimpanzees, which are kept in captivity and are fed a human type of food, never suffer from arteriosclerosis (calcification of the arteries) and never suffer from autoimmune diseases. However, elephants which are fed with grain and hay instead of their natural leaf diet, often suffer from blockages in their coronary arteries. Because chimpanzees do not possess this lectin-attaching sugar molecule, they do not suffer when they eat muesli, but humans and elephants can suffer from massive heart and autoimmune problems if we consume Lectins from grain.

WHAT HAPPENS IN OUR INTESTINES?

Lectins cannot be completely digested nor can they even be excreted, undigested, from the body. The low pH-value in the stomach does not affect the Lectins and they can pass into the intestines, where they are also able to resist the digestive enzymes. Here they can attach themselves to the cells of the mucous wall of the intestine and can be responsible for negatively influencing the balance of growth and replacement of these cells. This causes damage to the microvilli which are found in the intestine. These are filamentous protrusions on the intestinal mucosa which, in a healthy condition, increase the surface area of the intestines in order to achieve optimum nutritional absorption. If these are damaged, nutritional absorption and digestion become compromised. This is why they call Lectins anti-nutrition.

The changes in the cell metabolism of the intestinal wall (Epithelium) cause changes to the bacterial balance of the intestines (intestinal flora). Undigested food helps to increase the production of specific intestinal bacteria, leading to an over-production of these bacteria, in particular, E. coli (Escherichia coli).

This bacterium is not normally a problem for our health. However, an over-production causes an imbalance to occur.

WHAT HAPPENS OUTSIDE OUR INTESTINES?

The consumption of Lectins can cause an interaction with the enzymes in the body, which in turn, can adversely affect the digestion of proteins. Undigested Lectins can attach themselves to the cells on the intestinal walls which can enter the blood circulation and could consequently enter other internal organs. This can cause changes within the affected organs and the metabolism, resulting in the limitation of the body's own immune functions and capacity for growth.

I would like to point out that most studies were carried out using concentrated and isolated Lectins. However, we ingest a much lower concentration of Lectins with our diets and always in combination with other forms of nutrition. Because of this, it is not possible to connect directly the results of the studies with the way Lectins affect our diets.

The only substances which have been well researched up to now are the Lectins PHA (Phyto haemagglutinin) and WGA (wheat germ agglutinin) which can be found in raw kidney beans and wheat germ.

LECTINS CAUSING DISORDERS AND DISEASES

Many disorders and diseases can be linked to Lectins. We should also not underestimate the threat of Lectin poisoning from eating raw beans.

Not all Lectins cause poisoning. However, eating inadequately cooked kidney beans can lead to acute poisoning. The Lectin which is causing the trouble in this instance is phytohaemagglutinin (PHA). In the form of Phasin, this Lectin is mostly to be found in legumes, such as beans. The phytohaemagglutinin i.e. Phasin, is transmitted to the human organism through raw kidney beans, causing agglutination of the red blood corpuscles (Erythrocytes).

Symptoms of poisoning usually occur 2 to 3 hours after consumption. The seriousness of this poisoning varies significantly from person to person. It can cause nausea, abdominal discomfort and vomiting. The accompanying diarrhoea could be bloody. In addition to a fever, shivering and sweating, it can also cause cramps and shock.

On suspicion of poisoning, you should drink a lot of water. After consumption of larger, or unknown amounts, a doctor should be called immediately and detoxification should be carried out.

Poisoning can be avoided by sufficiently cooking the legumes in order to make the phytohaemagglutinin harmless.

The consumption of Lectins in large amounts can have consequences for our health and well-being. Discomfort and diseases originating from Lectins are often not recognised as being caused by them. The following is a list of symptoms which can be connected to high-Lectin nutrition:

- Joint pain
- Acid reflux
- Acne
- Aging spots
- Allergies
- Hair loss
- Skin problems, dermatitis, vitiligo
- Anaemia
- Arthritis
- Asthma
- Autoimmune diseases (diabetes Type I, Morbus Crohn, Lupus, Hashimoto)

- Osteoporosis
- Neuropathy
- Cancer
- Depression
- Dementia
- Exhaustion
- Headaches
- Migraine
- Tinnitus
- Dizziness
- Tooth decay
- Low testosterone values
- Weight problems

POSITIVE CHARACTERISTICS OF LECTINS

There are Lectins which are useful for human beings.

The Lectin in mistletoe (Viscum album L.), for example, can inhibit the growth of tumours. For this reason, it is used to support cancer therapies. In addition, it can stimulate the immune system by improving the production of cytokines and natural killer cells. The killer cells are responsible for recognising and killing tumour cells. They can be found in a medication called Lektinol, which can improve the general quality of life for cancer patients as well as improving their tolerance to conventional cancer therapy.

They are also relevant in the therapy of cardiovascular diseases and metabolic diseases as well as in combating the HI-Virus.

THE LEAKY GUT SYNDROME

The leaky gut syndrome is a barrier disorder of the small intestine. For various reasons, small holes develop in the intestinal wall. In this way, small amounts of toxins, pathogens and allergies can find their way into the body and cause inflammations, infections, allergies and, in the worst cases, autoimmune diseases.

Lectins play a significant role in the development of these syndromes, which is why I want to dedicate a part of my book to it. It is possible to diagnose and cure a leaky gut syndrome - here nutrition and lifestyle play a key role. Consuming a low-Lectin diet can help prevent or treat leaky gut syndrome.

HOW ARE THE BOWELS STRUCTURED?

The bowel is the largest organ in as far as surface area is concerned, although the heaviest organ is our skin, which has a surface area of 2m². In contrast to that, the complete, unfolded bowel would be equal to 180m², which is roughly the size of half a football field.

The bowel is only a few thousandths of a millimetre thick, only as thick as a single cell. Only a single cell separates the blood circulation from all the pathogens, toxins and nutrients in the bowel.

The cells in the bowel have the following functions:

- **Nutrient absorption:** Absorption of certain nutrients out of the food pulp (bolus).

- **Barrier:** Protective function against everything which should not enter the body. This includes bacteria, viruses, mould, worms, toxins and undigested proteins.

- **Immune System:** 70% of all immune cells in the body are located in the bowel. This makes sense because it is here that the greatest interaction with pathogens occurs.

- **Discharge:** Through bile salts and other mechanisms, toxins are discharged into the bowel in order to be released in the stools. The bowel plays an important role in cleansing the body.

- **Intestinal flora:** In the small intestine, there are only a few micro-organisms and bacteria. However, in the large intestine there are many more. In every drop of large intestinal fluid there are more living organisms than there are people on earth. We have many good bacteria in our large intestines and these are important to prevent pathogens and to break down undigested dietary fibre. The body profits from these metabolites and what the "good intestinal bacteria" produces: vitamins, messenger materials and healthy fats.

These functions are vital for humans. If the bowel becomes damaged, many important functions of the body would suffer. This works to the benefit of autoimmune diseases.

WHAT IS THE LEAKY GUT SYNDROME?

As previously mentioned, the bowel has a very large surface area, but it is wafer-thin, even thinner than a hair. A single cell protects your body from the micro-organisms in the bowel. If these should find their way out of the bowel, this could cause serious complications.

If the bowel ruptures, and these micro-organisms flow through the body unimpeded, a human could die within a few days from septicaemia. That is the worst-case scenario and is luckily very rare. It is much more probable that the bowel does not split extensively, but that many small holes appear, which brings us to the subject of this section – the leaky gut syndrome.

The bowel cells have an average lifespan of five days. The reason for this is that they are very active, metabolically, and are subject to a constant bombardment of pathogens. Because they are damaged so often, they need to be replaced quickly.

When the bowel has been strongly attacked, nutrition, which the cells need to replace themselves quickly, is in short supply. This causes the holes in the bowel. The bowel ceases to function as a filter and in particular areas is unable to prevent toxins and pathogens from reaching the blood circulation. These holes begin isolated and scattered but they can accumulate in the bowel, causing enormous damage to the body.

When holes in the bowel occur, we speak of "leaky gut syndrome".

These holes can also appear when the adhesion of the bowel cells tears apart. Normally the cells are firmly anchored. The proteins, which have a function in this process, are called "tight junctions". There are factors which can cause these junctions to split. These include, for example, Glutens (which we know belong to the Lectin group), which can also cause holes in the intestinal wall.

When the mucous layer becomes too thin, this poses a significant risk factor in the appearance of holes. The intestinal wall is covered by a thin mucous layer. This has the function of protecting the bowel cells from pathogens and to allowing the absorption of nutrients into the body. If this mucous layer becomes too thin, too weak or is besieged by anti-bacterial substances, direct contact occurs between the bowel cells and the intestinal flora. The intestinal wall could then be attacked by pathogens and, in the worst case, could cause the intestinal wall to split.

Very important: Once holes have appeared in the bowel, they have to be repaired and the bowel must be regenerated, as soon as possible in order to minimise damage.

HOW DO YOU RECOGNISE LEAKY GUT SYNDROME?

If you suffer from the following symptoms often, and for longer periods of time, the reason for your belly pain and digestion problems could be leaky gut syndrome:

- Irregular bowel movements which are too loose in consistency
- Frequent diarrhoea with occasional blood in the stools
- Flatulence
- Skin impurities
- Slightly puffy skin in the face
- Frequent allergic reactions and hay fevers
- Chronic fatigue, despite consuming sufficient food

In particular, irregular, inconsistent bowel movements with occasional blood is a direct marker, showing that there is damage to the bowel. If this is the case, I recommend being particularly attentive.

WHICH AUTOIMMUNE DISEASES DOES IT CAUSE?

If toxins, undigested proteins and pathogens are absorbed into the body, unimpeded, it can be dangerous and the chance of suffering the following side effects also increases:

- Hay fever and allergies
- Autoimmune diseases
- Chronic inflammation in the body
- Diabetes Type 2
- Blood poisoning
- Pancreatitis (inflammation of the pancreas)
- Hepatitis (inflammation of the liver)

In particular, the link to autoimmune disease has become more apparent in the last few years. There are signs that leaky gut syndrome can be linked to nearly every autoimmune disease. In the meantime, leaky gut syndrome is said to be one of the central causes in the emergence of autoimmune disease. This means, that the symptoms of autoimmune disease can be improved if the leaky gut syndrome can be healed.

HOW IS IT DIAGNOSED?

The patient's own documentation about his/her symptoms in the form of a symptom diary can be very useful to the doctor, or therapist, in forming a diagnosis. Most importantly, note should be taken when symptoms appear and how strongly they are felt. A report on your nutrition is also an important factor. Write down what you have eaten and drunk. It is equally important to record your bowel movements. All this information is important for a doctor or therapist to deliver the correct diagnosis.

WHO CAN DIAGNOSE A LEAKY GUT SYNDROME?

If you notice symptoms of leaky gut syndrome, you should visit a doctor quickly in order to obtain a diagnosis. This can be a general practitioner, a gastroenterologist, a homeopathic practitioner, a naturopath, an orthomolecular, mitochondrial or functional practitioner. These disciplines have the necessary knowledge and methods to recognise and treat a leaky gut syndrome.

In conventional medicine, leaky gut syndrome is not given as much importance, so I would recommend finding a doctor who combines conventional and natural medicine. This combination offers the best chances of diagnosis and treatment.

WHAT IS TESTED?

A diagnosis is determined when the following measurements are made and a positive result found:

Permeability test:

This test is based on the fact that certain sugars, normally from the intestines, are not absorbed. By leaky gut syndrome it can lead to sugars being absorbed involuntarily. The sugars used in these tests cannot be absorbed into the body and are excreted in the urine. If these sugars are found in the urine, a leaky gut syndrome can be diagnosed:

- Lactulose Mannitol test
- Lactulose Mannitol Glucose test
- 53Cr-EDTA test

Stool Sample:

A stool sample provides very valuable information for a diagnosis.

- Immune cells in the stool: With leaky gut syndrome immune cells can get into the inner bowel. These are then found in the stools.

- Calprotectin: This is a protein which can only be found in immune cells. If an immune cell is found in the stool, you will also be able to find Calprotectin.

- Lactoferrin: Similar to Calprotectin, Lactoferrin is also detectable in the stool.

- Blood can also be found in the stool.

- Secretory IgA: This antibody (Immunoglobulin) is produced in the Paneth cells of the intestinal wall and have an antibacterial effect. If there is a large amount in the stool, this suggests significant damage to the intestinal wall.

- α1-Anti-trypsin: This antibody is characteristic of leaky gut syndrome and if the condition is present it can be found in the stool.

- Zonulin: Not the most reliable marker but nevertheless is used frequently.

Blood test:

Leaky gut syndrome can also be diagnosed through a blood test:

- hsCRP: Universal inflammation marker which establishes if a chronic inflammation is present in the body.

- LPS (Lipopolysaccharide): If bacteria enter the blood circulation unimpeded, LPS can be found in the blood. LPS is a component of the bacterial cell wall. The body reacts particularly sensitively to LPS by causing inflammation. This can also be detected in the blood.

- LBP (LPS binding protein)

- α1-Anti-Trypsin: can be detected in the blood.

- TNFα: Another inflammation marker in the blood which is significantly increased in the presence of chronic infections and inflammations.

- sCD14

- I-FABP: (not very sensitive but widespread)

Using these markers, it is possible to detect leaky gut syndrome. Normally, it is better to measure too many, rather than too few of these markers. A large number of doctors resist these comprehensive tests because many of them (mostly conventional practitioners) do not recognise the term leaky gut syndrome. If the symptoms are very strong and last for a long time, you should insist that your doctor make these tests or perhaps you should look for another doctor. In an emergency, there is also the possibility of having testing done at your own expense. If there is compelling evidence of leaky gut syndrome, it is money well-spent because it can cause considerable damage to the body.

WHO TREATS THE LEAKY GUT SYNDROME?

Normally, the doctors who discover a leaky gut syndrome want to treat it themselves. Treatment differs, depending on how progressive your doctor is. I recommend changing your doctor if he prescribes Cortisone pain medicine, Mesalamine or antibiotics. These are all medicines which reduce the inflammation and immune reaction (or are supposed to treat an intestinal infection). However, this is counter-productive when treating a leaky gut syndrome, because there are other causes and it is only the symptoms which are being treated but not the healing of the intestine. Such treatments suggest a lack of knowledge about leaky gut syndrome by the doctor.

It is reckless to treat only the symptoms of leaky gut syndrome but not the cause. Here is a small example which illustrates this: Imagine you are standing for 24 hours with a bucket and cloth, trying to wipe away the water which is dripping into your home from a hole in the roof. If you do not repair the hole, you will be standing there for years, wiping away the water. The hole will grow bigger and bigger and wiping away the huge amount of water becomes increasingly exhausting. The size of the hole in the roof causes new dangers, as bugs and animals can enter into your house and cause damage of their own. This is roughly how your intestine behaves, if it is not treated.

WHAT SHOULD YOU BE AWARE OF WITH LEAKY GUT SYNDROME?

It is equally important to remove the causes of leaky gut syndrome as it is to patch up the holes.

Ideally you would be treated by a general practitioner, naturopath, alternative practitioner, orthomolecular or functional doctor. You can make the following statement about your treatment to yourself: You can recognise the effectiveness of the treatment by observing a decrease in the symptoms and an increase in your well-being.

Let us start with the causes: The following factors can trigger the leaky gut syndrome and exacerbate the symptoms. Try to create a healthier daily life and avoid the following things – or at least reduce them:

LECTINS

Lectins have played a central role in the emergence of leaky gut syndrome. This also the reason why I am so keen to state the connection between Lectins and leaky gut syndrome. I have already discussed how Lectins can cause damage to the intestines in the Chapter "What happens in our intestines?"

Gluten is one of the most important factors which can lead to leaky gut syndrome. It is the gluten in grain and can be found, for example in wheat, spelt, barley or rye. In sourdough products Gluten is not a problem, due to a fermentation process during production. However, sourdough products are more the exception than the rule.

In industrially processed bread, bakery products and pasta, gluten remains unchanged throughout the process. It is very difficult to digest and actively attacks the bonds between the intestinal cells, the so-called "tight junctions". This way, Gluten can directly cause holes in the intestines. Many people react adversely today by having a gluten intolerance.

For this reason, you should remove gluten-containing food completely from your diet and try to keep to gluten-free nutrition.

Oats and maize do not contain gluten but can also cause stomach irritation because of other Lectins. I also recommend avoiding these.

You should be aiming for a low-Lectin diet in order to achieve long-term improvement.

SUGAR

Industrial sugar in large amounts is not good for our intestines and can cause intolerance. The problem with sugar is the fructose (fruit sugar), which is a part of the household sugar.

This can also cause inflammatory reactions in the intestinal walls and facilitate the forming of holes. Try to reduce your sugar consumption to the minimum. Please note that many industrially-made products contain sugar. The best thing is to leave them out of your diet. You can reduce your sugar consumption and do something good for your intestines, particularly when you drink water instead of sweetened drinks.

FAST FOOD

Industrially prepared food contains many toxic additives and trans fats which can damage your intestinal wall. These additives cannot be found in nature. Our body is not used to them and they attack the intestinal wall directly.

I recommend avoiding all fast foods or industrially prepared foods, such as deep-frozen pizzas, biscuits, French fries, Peanut Flips and ice cream. If a food contains ingredients which you cannot understand without a Chemistry degree, it is better not to touch them, because they are damaging to the intestines.

ALCOHOL

Similar to sugar, alcohol can directly cause inflammation of the intestines. If your intestines are already damaged, it is advisable to greatly reduce your alcohol intake.

SPORT

People who do competitive sports put their intestines under pressure. The continual mechanical shocks to the body and the low blood circulation of the intestines can lead to leaky gut syndrome. This pertains particularly to competitive sports. Those who participate in normal sporting activities are improving their health and it is important to understand the difference. I am not saying that you should not participate in sporting activity. If you are suffering from inflammation of the intestinal mucosa, it would be advisable to reduce the amount of sport you are doing, or change to a lighter form of sport, in order to allow your intestines to return to normal. Once the inflammation has healed, you can resume gentle physical activity.

STRESS

The body releases the stress hormone, Cortisol, if it is subject to chronic stress. This hormone gives you the energy to cope with the stress situation. Stress in everyday life and at work causes a continual excess in the production of Cortisol. The problem with this hormone is that it prevents the growth of intestinal cells. Too much stress often means holes in the intestines. For this reason, it is essential to actively reduce the amount of stress you are subject to.

FOOD ALLERGENS

If the proteins in your food are not completely digested, they can access your blood circulation, as in the case of leaky gut syndrome. As a result, the body's immune system produces antibodies. This, in turn, causes food allergies of varying degrees. It does not have to be a strong reaction, it can be subtle and hidden. It could show itself, for example, in blemished skin, chronic exhaustion or hay fever.

Inflammation caused by food allergies can lead to leaky gut syndrome. Ask your doctor to perform a food allergy test.

MEDICATIONS

Much too often, antibiotics are prescribed, although they are not necessary. Antibiotics can save lives in the case of life-threatening infections caused by bacteria but not by virus infections or intestinal problems. Antibiotics kill everything in the intestines. That means that the bad intestinal bacteria are eliminated but also the good ones which are important for the intestinal flora. This makes the problem worse.

You should only take antibiotics if a bad infection is present, which the doctor confirms cannot be treated any other way.

Due to their way of working, non-steroid anti-inflammatory drugs, better known as pain killers, can cause small amounts of bleeding in the intestines. If you take painkillers or blood thinners, such as Aspirin, Ibuprofen or Diclophenac, over a long period of time, this can also be the cause of a leaky gut syndrome.

DIET FOR LEAKY GUT SYNDROME

When considering your diet, it is important to avoid the risk factors for irritation of the intestines. This means avoiding Lectins, sugar, fast foods and alcohol. There are some known nutritional concepts which take this into consideration. In the next chapter I will introduce you to Gundry's nutritional concept, which focuses on low-Lectin consumption.

It is important to see this as a long-term change in diet, otherwise the intestines will only settle for a short time after which the symptoms will return.

In order to regenerate the intestinal flora, it is useful to make a kind of fasting. Gundry's nutritional concept is divided into three phases. In the first phase, only the most digestible foods are consumed, which do not irritate the gastrointestinal tract and which allow the development of new intestinal flora.

FOOD SUPPLEMENTS AND NUTRIENTS FOR LEAKY GUT SYNDROME.

Once you have been diagnosed with leaky gut syndrome, you can choose from several food supplements which have been tried and tested. People who have been watching their diet and keeping to the plan should be able to take sufficient quantities of these vitamins and minerals in their nutrition. However, a doctor or therapist may recommend the following additives in order to support the regeneration process.

- Vitamin D (Target value in blood: 60-80 ng/ml, rule of thumb: 1000 I.U. Vitamin D per 10 ng/ml vitamin deficiency). The blood values should be determined by the doctor.

- Glutamine (for intestinal regeneration 20–30 g daily for two weeks)

- Bone broth (one glass daily)

- N-Acetyl-Cysteine (usual daily dose 2–3 g)

- Curcumin (500-1000 mg daily)

- Omega 3 fatty acids 8.17 / fish oil capsules (on the days when you do not eat fish, it is recommended to take 3-5 g Omega 3 fatty acids in the form of fish oil capsules)

DIET WITHOUT LECTINS

THE GUNDRY THEORY

Dr. Gundry is the pioneer or the father of low- Lectin nutrition. With self-experiments and research with his patients, he has developed many theories, and has a lot of experience, on the subject of Lectins. His book is a best-seller and his name appears immediately as soon as you research the subject of Lectins. Also, my literature is based on the experiments of Gundry who laid the foundations for a low-Lectin way of eating. As a result of his many successes in the treatment of patients, using his recommended diets, he gives hope in the treatment of all disorders and diseases.

ABOUT STEVEN R. GUNDRY

Dr. Steven R. Gundry is an American doctor and author. He is a former cardiac surgeon and currently runs his own clinic, purportedly investigating the impact of diet on health. Gundry conducted cardiology research in the 1990s and was a pioneer in infant heart transplant surgery, and is a New York Times best-selling author of books such as "*The Plant Paradox: The Hidden Dangers in "Healthy" Foods That Cause Disease and Weight Gain.*"

Gundry carried out nutritional trials on himself in order to test the impact of Lectins on health. He ate wholemeal muesli and a lot of fruit and vegetables. He began to suffer from arthritis and high blood pressure, his sugar and cholesterol values rose and he put on a lot of weight.

SUCCESS IN THE TREATMENT OF DISEASES

Since he began his research, Dr. Gundry reports that he has treated more than 1000 patients. With his diet, he had found a method to save some patients the trauma of a heart operation.

In his book he gives several examples of successfully treated patients with their symptoms.

Yvonne (50):	Serious Lupus with joint pain, fatigue and rashes
Suzanna (27):	Very pronounced rheumatic arthritis (desire to have children)
Vegan Cookbook author (81):	Serious arthritis, Lupus, Celiac disease (Inflammation of the mucous membrane of the small intestine)
Jill (20):	Crohn's disease
Michael (13):	Crohn's disease
Jennifer (71):	Rheumatoid arthritis
Sara (71):	Strong abdominal pain, joint pain, arthritis
Emily:	Raynaud syndrome

	(autoimmune disease)
Japanese sculptor (77):	Serious Arthritis
Maria (47):	Diabetes
Marcia (29):	MS
Simon (40):	Alzheimer Gene
Molly (74):	Fatty liver, diabetes
Jane (50):	Serious migraine
Patrick (40):	Chronic fatigue syndrome
Amelia (51):	Diabetes, high blood pressure, high cholesterol values

LIST OF FOODS

Gundry has two food lists, one for positive foods which are low in Lectins and the other is the negative food list which shows foods which are high in Lectins. The idea is to orientate yourself on the positive list and cut out the foods on the negative one.

POSITIVE FOODS

In the food list, there are various numbers with specific meanings. These are important to note when changing your diet.

Here is the explanation:

- [1] = recommended in the first 3 days (Phase 1)
- [2] = recommended in the first 6 weeks (Phase 2)
- [3] = Keto-Intensive programme for serious illnesses
- [33] = more valuable than [3]
- * = only with pressure cooker

Oils:

- Linseed oil [1 2 3]
- Walnut oil [1 2 3]
- Shiso oil (Perilla) [1 2 33]
- Hemp oil [1 3]
- Camelina oil [1 2 3]
- Cedar oil [1 2 3]
- Olive oil [33]
- Coconut oil [33]
- Macadamia oil [1 2 33]
- MCT oil [1 2 33]
- Avocado oil [1 2 3]
- Algae oil [1 2 3]
- Sesame oil [1 3]
- Red Palm oil [3]
- Rice bran oil [3]
- Cod liver oil [2 3]

- Omega 3 Fisch oil capsules [2,3]

Sweeteners:
- Stevia /leaves [1,3]
- Yacon [3]
- Honey (max 1 tsp/day)
- Inulin [1,3]
- Luo han guo [3]
- Erythritol [3]
- Xylitol [3]

Vegetables:
- Broccoli [1,2,3]
- Brussel Sprouts [1,2,3]
- Cauliflower [1,2,3]
- Pak Choi [1,2,3]
- Chinese cabbage [1,2,3]
- Cabbage Kale [1,2,3]
- Chard [1,2,3]
- Spinach [1,2,3]
- Kohlrabi [1,2,3]
- White and red cabbage [1,2,3]
- Radicchio [1,2,3]
- Raw Sauerkraut [1,2,3]
- Onions [1,2,3]
- Garlic [1,2,3]
- Artichokes [1,2,3]
- Chicory [1,2,3]
- Nettle [1,2,3]
- Bull rush pulp [1,2,3]
- Willow herb leaves [1,2,3]
- Gout weed [1,2,3]
- Linden leaves [1,2,3]
- Comfrey
- Hogweed
- Leek [1,3]
- Chives [1,3]
- Spring onion [1,3]
- Watercress [1,3]
- Radish [1,3]

- Coriander [1] [3]
- Asparagus [1] [3]
- Romaine lettuce [1] [3]
- Celery [1] [3]
- green and red leaf salad [1] [3]
- Baby lettuce leaves [1] [3]
- Fennel [1] [3]
- Parsley [1] [3]
- Basil [1] [3]
- Mint [1] [3]
- Rocket [1] [3]
- Jerusalem artichoke [2] [3]
- Okra [2] [3]
- Mushrooms [2] [3]
- Endives [2] [3]
- Chicory [3]
- Raw carrots [3]
- Carrot greens [3]
- Beetroot [3]
- Daikon radish [3]
- Milk sour vegetables [3]
- Dandelion [3]
- Lettuce [3]
- Mustard leaves [3]
- Mizuna Turnip greens [3]
- Purslane [3]
- Shiso [3]
- Algae (Nori) [1] [3]
- Seaweed (Kelp) [1] [3]
- Cactus fruit (prickly pear) [3]
- Palm hearts [3]
- Legumes*
- Chickpeas*
- Hummus*
- Lentils*
- Broad beans*

Grazing animals - Poultry:

(120gr per day)

(60 bis 120gr per day) [3]

- Grazing animal - eggs (up to 4 per day) [2]
(up to 4 egg yolks + 1 Egg white) [3]
- Chicken [1]
- Turkey [3]
- Duck [3]
- Goose [3]
- Pheasant [3]
- Pidgeon [3]
- Quail [3]
- Grouse [3]
- Ostrich [3]

Pasta:

- Pasta slim [3]
- Shirataki noodles [3]
- Kelp Noodles [3]
- Miracle noodles [3]
- Sweet potato noodles [3]

Herbs and Spices:

All [1,2,3] except Chili Pepper

- Mustard [1,2,3]
- fresh black Pepper [1,2,3]
- Sea salt [1,2,3]
- Miso [3]

Flour:

- Almond [3]
- Hazelnut [3]
- Chestnut [3]
- Tiger nut [3]
- Grape seed [3]
- Sweet potato [3]
- Linseed [3]
- Cedar nut [3]

- Coconut [3]
- Sesame [3]
- Manioc [3]

- Green banana [3]
- Arrowroot [3]

Nuts and seeds:
(1/2 cup per day)
- Walnut [1 2 33]
- Hazelnut [1 3]
- Chestnut [1 3]
- Linseed [1 3]
- Hemp seed [1 33]
- Hemp protein powder [1 33]
- Pine nut (few) [1]
- Cedar nut [1]
- Beech nut almond [1]

[3]
- Macadamia [1 2 33]
- Pistachio [1 2 3]
- Pecan [1 3]
- Coconut (not coconut water) [1 3]
- Coconut milk [1 3]
- Brazil nut (few) [1 3]
- Psyllium [1 3]
- Sesame [1 3]

Milk products:
(30 g cheese or 120 g yoghurt per day)
- Goatmilk and cream, goat and sheep butter [3]
- Goat and sheep cheese [3]
- Goat and sheep yoghurt, goat and sheep Kefir [3]
- Butter [33]
- Ghee [2 33]
- Casein A2 milk as cream, Casein A2

- cheese bio-confectioners cream (cream with 35-40% Fat) [3]
- Sour cream [3]
- Whey protein powder, double cream cheese (Philadelphia)
- Ghee [33]
- Real Parmesan (Parmigiano Reggiano)
- Real Pecorino
- French / Italian Butter [33]
- Coconut yoghurt [3]
- French / Italian cheese
- Swiss cheese
- Extra fat cheese from F/I/CH [3]
- Ghee (Italian) [3]

Wine:

(170ml/day) red [3]

Grain:
- Millet [2,3]
- Sorghum [2,3]
- white Basmati Rice (little)*

Resistant Starch:

(in moderate amounts)
- Tubers, celery [1,2,3]
- Yams [2,3]
- Turnip [2,3]
- Parsnip [2,3]
- Yucca blossom [2,3]

- Konjac tuber [2,3]
- Persimmon [2,3]
- Brassica [2,3]
- Tiger nut [2,3]
- Millet [2,3]
- Sorghum [2,3]
- Sweet potato [2,3]
- Plantain [2,3]
- Green banana [2,3]
- Baobab fruit [2,3]
- Tapioca [2,3]
- Yam bean [2,3]
- Taro root [2,3]
- Green Mango [2,3]
- Green Papaya [2,3]

Drinks:

- Water (Spring or filtered) [1,2,3]
- Herb tea [1,2,3]
- Green tea [1,2,3]
- Black tea [1,2,3]
- Coffee (with or without caffeine) [1,2,3]

Fish:

Wild caught fish only (120 gr per day) [2] (60 to 120 gr per day including meat) [3]

- White fish (Vendace / carp) [1,2,33]
- Mussels [1,2,33]
- Mackerel [1,2,33]
- Herring [1,2,33]
- Trout [1,2,33]
- Alaska Halibut [1,2,33]
- Tuna fish [1,33]
- Alaska Salmon [1,2,33]
- Prawns [1,2,33]
- Shrimps [1,2,33]
- Lobster [1,2,33]

- Octopus [1 2 33]
- Oysters [1 2 33]
- Sardines [1 2 33]
- Anchovies [1 2 33]

Fruit:

(apart from Avocado all limited)

- Bilberry
- Raspberry
- Blackberry
- Strawberry
- Blackcurrant
- Gooseberry
- Grape
- Rock pear
- Honey berry
- Cornelian cherry
- Oleaster
- Mulberry
- Cherry
- Pear
- Pomegranate
- Kiwi
- Apple
- Nectarine
- Peach
- Plum
- Apricot
- Fig [2]
- Cherry plum
- Pawpaw
- Korea cherry
- Medlar
- Sea buckthorn
- Hawthorn
- Quince
- Avocado [1 3]
- Citrus (no juice)
- Lemon juice [1 2]
- Dates [2]

Olives [3]:

all

Dark Chocolate:
72% or more (30gr / day)
90% or more (30gr / day) [3]

Vinegar [1] [2] [3]:
All without added sugar

Meat from Grazing Animals:
(120 gr per day)
(60 to 120 gr per day incl. fish) [3]

- Pork [3]
- Lamb [3]
- Game [3]
- Venison [3]
- Wild boar [3]
- Beef [3]
- Bison [3]
- Prosciutto ham

Plant-based „meat":
- Quorn (gluten free mushroom sporn)
- Hemp-Tofu [1] [3]
- Tempeh (only grain-free) [1] [3]

---

[1] Additions by Konstantin Kirsch from the book „The Plant Paradox" by Dr. Steven Gundry, pages 201-203 / 262-265 incl. several notes in the text. No liability assumed.

NEGATIVE FOODS

Dr. Gundry said: "RULE NUMBER 1: What you stop eating has far more impact on your health than what you start eating."

Every food which is marked with a star (*) is allowed in phase 2. However, these foods should be prepared properly and cooked in a pressure cooker.

Refined Starchy Foods

- Pasta
- Rice
- Potatoes
- Potato crisps
- Milk
- Bread
- Tortillas
- Pastries
- Flour
- Cereals
- Muesli
- Sugar
- Agave
- Acesulfame K
- Sucralose
- Aspartame
- Saccharin
- Maltodextrin
- Diet drinks

Vegetables:

- Peas
- Mangetout pea
- Pea protein
- Green beans
- All beans incl. shoots

- Legumes *
- Chickpeas *
- Hummus *
- Lentils *
- Edamame (unripe soy beans)
- Soy protein
- Textured plant protein

Fruit:

- Cucumber
- Zucchini
- Pumpkin (all sorts)
- Melon (all sorts)
- Eggplant
- Tomato
- Bell pepper
- Broad beans *
- Soy
- Tofu
- Chili
- Goji berry

Non-south European milk Products:

(these contain Casein-A1)

- Yoghurt (incl. Greek Yoghurt)
- Ice cream
- Yoghurt ice cream

Nuts and Seeds

- Pumpkin
- Sunflower

- Chia seeds

Oils
- Sunflower oil
- Cheese
- Ricotta
- Cottage Cheese
- Rapeseed oil
- Corn oil
- Peanut oil
- Thistle oil
- Grape seed oil

- Peanut
- Cashew
- Soy bean oil
- Vegetable oil (Pseudonym for Soy oil)
- Partly hardened oil

Grain, Pseudo-grain, Sprouts and Grasses

- Wheat

   (pressure cooking does not remove Lectins from any grain type)

- Einkorn
- Kamut ®

- Oat
- Quinoa
- Rye
- Bulgur
- White rice
- Brown rice

- Wild rice
- White Basmati rice*
- Barley
- Buckwheat
- Spelt
- Corn

- Corn products
- Corn starch
- Corn syrup
- Wheat grass
- Barley grass

---

[2] Additions to the Book "The Plant Paradox" by Dr. Steven Gundry made by Konstantin Kirsch

CASEIN A2 MILK

There is a wide range of milk variations. This includes raw milk, homogenised milk and also reduced-fat H-milk. Everyone has his/her own favourite, mostly governed by the taste or the fat content.

Something which is not so well-known is that there is another difference in milk types; A1 and A2 milk, the latter being "natural whole milk", the original milk from the refrigerated section, but why is it hard to find this milk, these days?

WHAT IS THE DIFFERENCE BETWEEN A1 AND A2 MILK?

The answer is: Proline instead of Histidine. There is a small difference in the amount of amino acids they contain.

To understand better the difference, we have to understand the composition of milk. Apart from a lot of water, milk contains fat and proteins. The protein mainly to be found in milk is Casein. There are different kinds of Casein, including Beta-Casein, which is made of 209 amino acids. The difference between A1 and A2 milk is at position 67 of this chain of amino acids. In A2 Beta-Casein, there is an amino acid called Proline, whereas in this place in A1, Histidine can be found.

WHAT HAPPENS DURING DIGESTION OF A1 MILK?

This subtle difference has a great impact on digestion and health. During digestion, a chain of amino acids is broken down creating opiate Beta-Casomorphin-7 (BCM7). This is not the case with A2 milk.

BCM7 causes several things to happen in the body. Firstly, it affects the opioid receptors in the digestive tract and the immune system. It can slow down digestion and cause constipation. In addition, it has been proved to cause a negative reaction to the development of new-born babies and small children, and by some children it has become apparent that BCM7 increases the risk factor for apnoea (respiratory arrest). There is also convincing evidence of a connection between BCM7 and the occurrence of coronary heart diseases and Diabetes Type 1.

Interestingly, pasteurising milk products increases the negative aspects. A1 milk is much richer in Lectins than A2 milk.

WHY IS THERE A DIFFERENCE BETWEEN A1 AND A2 MILK?

Originally all cows produced A2 milk. Due to a gene mutation, Europeans preferred the cattle breed which proved to have Histidine in their amino acid chain. Over the years, this led to an almost complete cessation in A2 milk producing cows. Today, in Europe, there are almost exclusively only cattle breeds which produce A1 milk.

WHY IS THIS NOT WELL-KNOWN?

There has not been much research in this area. Although in the last 10 to 15 years, research has intensified, there is still a lot of work to do. Current knowledge does seem to support the fact that A1 milk is not good for human health.

The milk industry has no great interest in reducing milk consumption. A changeover to A2 milk would cause immense costs. However, in this area, New Zealand is making a good example. In an important research project, herds were changed to those producing A2 milk with the aim of changing over completely to A2 milk within the next 10 years.

WHERE DO I FIND A2 MILK PRODUCTS?

The majority of the European and American cattle breeds belong to the sub-species "Bos primigenius taurus". Most of these animals produce A1 milk. An exception to this is the breed called "Jersey" which produces partly A1 and partly A2 milk and "Guernsey", which produces exclusively A2 milk.

Commercial milk usually comes from breeds such as "Holstein", which mainly produce A1 milk.

Those who would like to consume mainly A2 milk should find farmers which have "Guernsey" cattle for milk production. An alternative is the sub-species "Bos primigenius indicus" which is to be found on the sub-continent of Africa. Animals of this sub-species mostly produce A2 milk but are not very common in our latitudes. This makes A2 milk quite hard to find. It would be easier to search for goats, sheep, yaks or buffalo, which mostly produce A2 milk. Buffalo mozzarella, for example, is a good substitute for commercial mozzarella because it is made from pure A2 milk.

MAKING LECTINS HARMLESS

The list of high-Lectin foods is long. If you avoid all of them, it would be very difficult to cover your nutritional needs. The good news is that there are ways to significantly reduce the Lectins, if not completely eliminate them. Correct preparation is essential. However, the maximum nutrient content is useless if the food does not taste good. If you do not eat it, then you do not consume any nutrients. It is just as useless to aim for maximum nutritional content, if the effort is too high in achieving it. Cooking methods, such as steeping or fermentation can change the taste, e.g. make it taste stronger. I personally like that, but it is a question of personal taste and is not everyone's thing. So, I recommend to view everything in proportion and to find out for yourself what you like and what type of preparation does not suit you.

COOKING FOR LONG ENOUGH

Cooking legumes and rice for long enough is particularly important. The time should not fall below 15 minutes, preferably longer, in order to ensure that the Lectins have been reduced. It is particularly important with beans in order to destroy the toxins.

PEELING AND CORE REMOVAL

Usually, most Lectins are to be found in the peelings, the core or the seeds. Therefore, you should peel and core vegetables or fruit before consumption. This is also true of nuts. If you are sensitive to Lectins, it is possible for you to eat peeled almonds but not those with skin.

Also, high-Lectin vegetables, such as pumpkin, tomato, paprika or courgettes can be consumed if they are skinned by people who are not sensitive to Lectins.

STEEPING

In order to explain the principle of steeping, we first have to understand what happens to the plant. Steeping causes these plant embryos (grain and beans) to be in contact with water for a significant amount of time, as if they have been lying in the rain. That signals to the plant that it can commence growth. The plant begins to reduce its protective mechanisms and prepares to germinate. The Lectins reduce and the nutrients become more accessible. In order to obtain this result, it is advisable to steep grain and legumes before consumption. In today's western civilisation, hardly anyone does this. For this reason, an increasing number of people suffer from digestive diseases and grain is becoming tolerated by fewer people.

Generally, the steeping of grain, legumes and nuts works in the same way. Add water and wait 12 to 24 hours.

This is how you steep legumes: Place the beans or lentils in a glass, porcelain or ceramic bowl. Add three times the mass of lukewarm water i.e. 1.5 litre of water to 500 grams of beans. Allow to steep for 12 to 24 hours at room temperature. Discard the steeping water and cook the legumes in fresh water. It is important to note that the cooking time for these items will be reduced, due to the steeping. This way, you save energy and money. I do this with all legumes (peas, beans, lentils). You can change the water if you want, but it is not necessary because you could lose even more nutrients, which we want to eat. You could use the water used to steep the legume in for cooking because you pour away that water in the end anyway. During the warmer months, I only steep for 12 hours to prevent the legume from germinating.

This is how you steep grain: Put the grain (whole grains or ground) in a glass, porcelain or ceramic bowl. I choose the amount of water, depending on the eventual use of the grain. For porridge, I put five times the amount of water onto the ground oats, e.g. 300 millilitres of lukewarm water onto 60 grams of oatmeal. I cook the oats in the same water. For whole grains, I need less water. Three times the amount is enough in this instance. Then steep the grains for 12 to 24 hours at room temperature. Depending on what you are making, you can either pour away or keep the steeping water. Remember that here, too, the amount of cooking time is reduced due to the steeping process.

This will also save energy and money. Ready! I carry out the same process for all types of grain. As with legume, I do not rinse the corn or change the water, in order to retain the nutrients.

There are instructions for steeping which recommend the addition of acids, such as whey, yoghurt or lemon juice, and alkalis, such as baking soda. You can do this in order to influence the effect of the steeping. However, this changes the taste, which I, personally, do not like. You can try it and see which method you prefer.

By the way, beans from a jar or tin do not need to be cooked, they are already Lectin-free.

FERMENTING

Grinding the germinating grain increases the surface area considerably. This releases enzymes which perform important functions as described below. Using lactic acid (one spoonful of natural yoghurt can work wonders), Phytase begins to break down the phytic acid and making the grain a wonderful source of minerals. This is of course dependent on the type of grain. Corn, rice, oats and millet contain only a small amount of Phytase and therefore need a longer period of fermentation. The addition of other grain types, such as wheat, rye or buckwheat, whose Phytase content is relatively high, can help in the fermentation. This process also helps to make the Lectins less harmful and the amino acid profile changes, making the grain protein value similar to that of meat. At the same time, the digestibility of the grain increases so that these nutrients can penetrate better into the system. One form of fermentation in Europe is known as leavening. None of these processes have an appreciable influence on the effect of glutens in the digestive tract. However, there is evidence that our intestinal bacteria are better able to digest glutens which have undergone the fermentation process.

When it comes to soy, the fermented product called Tempeh is one of the few soy products, which is recognised as a positive food. Miso, a Japanese paste, which is mainly made from soy beans combined with a range of other food, such as rice, barley etc., or pseudo-grains and table salt, is a low-Lectin product. The Lectins in soy bean agglutinin (SBA) and soy bean Lectin (SBL) can only be eliminated through the fermentation process. All other soy products, such as tofu, have a very high Lectin content, which cannot be minimised sufficiently through other cooking methods.

Sourdough is another example of a fermented product which makes consumption safe, partly by deactivation of the Lectins. Naturally, we can ferment every kind of vegetable, thereby increasing their usefulness as far as health is concerned.

Here are some examples how you can ferment vegetables yourself and what you need for it.

I take the following ingredients:

- 2.6 lb Chinese cabbage
- 2 cloves of garlic

- 0.8 – 1.2 in piece of ginger
- 2 whole chilis
- 2 carrots
- 0.8 oz sea salt without additives (per 3.5 oz vegetable 0.7 oz salt)

Separate the leaves of Chinese cabbage and wash them. Cut them into rough pieces. Cut the carrots into fine strips and the garlic into slices. Peel and grate the ginger. Mix everything together in a large bowl and rub in the salt until liquid appears in the cabbage. Press the mass into a clean glass jar. It is important to press in well so that the vegetables are completely covered by the liquid.

Other vegetables can be fermented just as easily. Those vegetables which cannot be fermented in their own juices, such as carrots, sweet pepper, cauliflower, garlic or ginger can be pressed into a brine mixture which is made the following way:

Mix 2 cupful of water with 0.7 oz sea salt (without additives). At first, use a little hot water to dissolve the salt. Then add the rest of the cold water and fill the jar with the vegetables and cover with the liquid.

During fermentation, gases are created which pressurise the jar. I recommend, therefore, to use jars with a clip lock as they allow excess pressure to be released.

I would also always put the jars on a steel tray to catch any leakage. The fermentation takes 5-7 days at room temperature and, if possible, away from light. Once the fermentation process is complete, the jars are best kept in the refrigerator or cellar.

COOKING IN THE PRESSURE COOKER

Use a pressure cooker, or preferably a steam pressure cooker as Lectins are neutralised most effectively with the steam variation. This practical kitchen utensil could be a worthwhile investment. Above all, I found multi-purpose pressure cookers in which, for example, you can cook rice, to be very useful in the kitchen, because they can be used for various things.

The pressure and high temperature make the Glycoproteins harmless, particularly in potatoes and grain.

In a study, the Phytic acid content from steeped peas, cooked in a steam pressure cooker were compared to the normal preparation of these vegetables. With the peas, which had been cooked in a steam pressure cooker, there was a 54% reduction in Phytic acid content compared to 29% with normal cooking.

In addition, the steam pressure cooker had a further advantage compared to other methods of preparation in that nutrients were better preserved with this type of cooking.

FURTHER TIPS FOR EVERY DAY

AVOID HIGH-LECTIN FOODS

Unfortunately, there is no way around it but to avoid high-Lectin foods. Because Lectins can be found in almost all plant-based foodstuffs, it is almost impossible to avoid them. The first step is to eliminate the worst culprits. We can begin by excluding the following foods completely from our nutrition:

- Corn
- Meat from corn-fed animals. This includes most meat types which are sold in the food stores.
- Casein-A1 milk. Casein A2 is the normal protein from the milk which can be found in sheep, goats, water buffalo and some cow milk from Jersey. Unfortunately, most cows are Casein-A1 producers.
- Peanuts, cashews and non-fermented soy products. If you want to eat soy, make sure that is fermented in the traditional way, as in Tempeh.

ENJOY HIGH-LECTIN FOODS SPARINGLY

The following foods also contain Lectins. However, you can choose either to avoid them completely or eat them sparingly. I would like to remind you that correct preparation and cooking makes a big difference. Research shows that fermentation, steeping and cooking foods with high-Lectin content can reduce the Lectins so much that most people can eat them without problem.

- Legumes (plant seeds in pods, such as peas and beans)
- Grains, particularly wholemeal grain
- Nightshade fruits and vegetables (such as tomatoes, potatoes, aubergines, peppers and goji berries, just to mention a few)
- Cucurbit family fruits, such as pumpkin and courgette.

The Lectin content varies depending on the fruit/vegetable. There are bean types with less Lectins, such as rice beans, cowpeas, broad beans, lupin seeds,

Great Northern beans and Pinto Group III beans. Among the mid to low-content vegetables, and therefore the safest, are the Polish pea sorts and lentils. White kidney beans and soy beans belong to the high or middle Lectin-containing fruits/vegetables. Red kidney beans belong to the group which has the highest Lectin content of all. It is best to avoid these, especially if you are intolerant to Lectins or have a sickness which requires a low-Lectin diet.

In comparison: White kidney beans contain a third of the haem-agglutinating units of toxic Phyto-haem-agglutins compared to red kidney beans. Cowpeas contain only 5 to 10 percent of the Lectins.

THIS IS HOW YOU OPTIMISE THE HEALTH BENEFITS OF POTATOES.

Potatoes belong to the nightshade group of plants, which contain Lectins. The Lectin content can be reduced by cooking, although these Lectins are usually more heat-proof than beans. Cooking reduces the Lectin content by 50 to 60 percent. If you cool potatoes after they are cooked, you can increase the nutritional value of them. Cooling them increases the digestive-resistant starches in the potato fibres. This starch passes through the small intestine undigested and begins to ferment in the colon, causing bacteria to form which strengthen the intestinal flora.

For example, roasted and cooled potatoes contain 19 grams of resistant starch per 100 grams. Steamed and cooled potatoes only contain 6 grams. Boiled and cooled potatoes, however, contain only 0.8 grams.

SAFE LECTINS

Among the safest plant-based foods are asparagus, garlic, celery, mushrooms and onions. Other examples of excellent food, which you can eat without limit are:

- Boiled tubers (root vegetables), such as sweet potatoes, yucca and taro

- Leafy greens

- Cruciferous vegetables, such as broccoli, cauliflower and Brussel sprouts

- Avocados

- Olives and genuine native olive oil extra

WHITE GRAIN INSTEAD OF BROWN

Today it is assumed that brown grain is better than white. Gundry contradicts that completely. If you see it from the Lectins point of view, it makes a lot of sense to give preference to white rice and white bread. If you want to follow a low-Lectin diet, it is important to ensure that the bread is baked by traditional methods, best of all is sourdough bread.

Ensure that the grain is organically cultivated.

CHANGING YOUR DIET, STEP BY STEP

In the following, you will see how to change your diet permanently in three steps. Gundry speaks of the three phases. The first days are spent cleansing and regulating the intestinal flora. After that the focus is on choosing foods from the positive foods list and avoiding resolutely the negative foods. In phase 3, small amounts of high-Lectin foods can be tried out.

PHASE 1: CLEANSING/RESTORATION

Gundry says of the first phase: "Just as a gardener or farmer prepares the soil before planting"

In the next three days, you will prepare your body for the change in diet and cleanse your intestines.

In order to simplify the first three days, you can simply follow the eating plan given below. You will find all the recipes in the appropriate chapters.

FOOD PLAN FOR 3 DAYS:

Day 1

<u>Breakfast:</u>

Green smoothie

<u>Snack:</u>

Romaine lettuce boats filled with guacamole

<u>Lunch:</u>

Rocket salad with chicken and lemon vinaigrette

<u>Snack:</u>

Cabbage crisps

<u>Dinner:</u>

Cabbage-kale sauté with salmon and avocado*

Day 2

Breakfast:

Green smoothie

Snack:

Romaine lettuce boats filled with guacamole

Lunch:

Romaine salad with avocado and basil pesto chicken*

Snack:

Cabbage crisps

Dinner:

Lemony Brussel sprouts, kale and onions with cabbage "steak.

Day 3

<u>Breakfast:</u>

Green smoothie

<u>Snack:</u>

Romaine lettuce boats filled with guacamole

<u>Lunch:</u>

Asia wrap with chicken and coriander dip*

<u>Snack:</u>

Cabbage crisps

<u>Dinner:</u>

Roasted broccoli with cabbage rice and sautéed onions

Those meals which are marked with an asterisk (*) can be substituted with other vegetarian or vegan products. In the recipe section you can find the reference to that with suggestions for alternative variations.

In Gundry's food plan there is a recommendation for two snacks per day of "Romaine lettuce boats filled with guacamole". For me, personally, this is too much avocado. This is the reason I have substituted one snack with cabbage crisps.

For those who do not find cabbage crisps in the afternoon filling enough, I recommend preparing a double portion of guacamole in the morning and storing this in a covered bowl in the refrigerator. You can then use it as a dip for the cabbage chips.

Notice that sometimes the same recipe is used for the dressing of other dishes. Therefore, it can be time-saving to prepare two portions of the dressing, keeping the remainder in a glass jar to use in another meal the following day.

The chicken should not be from a feedlot or factory farming facility, where the animals are fed with antibiotics, corn, soy etc. Also, the fish should be wild-caught and may not be taken from a factory farming source. If it is not possible to obtain these, I recommend choosing a vegetarian substitute for them.

You may experience hunger during these three days because your digestion is used to another kind of diet. Keep persevering with the recommended snacks and, above all, drink a lot of water. I was able to tide myself over with water. This way you have something in your stomach and, at the same time, regenerating and washing the toxins out of your body.

Again, here is a short summary of what is permitted during the first days.

1. No more food which will burden your digestive system:

    Avoid: Milk and milk products, grain, fruit, sugar, eggs, soy, nightshade fruits and vegetables, root vegetables or large amounts of oil or meat.

    Use instead: vegetables, fish, proteins, hemp tofu, fats (avocado, olives) oils (avocado oil, coconut oil, walnut oil, sesame oil, olive oil, hempseed oil).

2. Snacks: Romaine lettuce boats with guacamole and cabbage chips.

3. Salad dressing: Fresh lemon, vinegar, freshly milled pepper, sea salt, herbs.

4. Drinks: Green smoothie, filtered water, green and black herb teas.

Positive effects on your body and mind after three days:

- Absolute positive balance in the intestinal bacteria

- Almost certain loss of weight of around 1.5 to 3 kg (mainly water)

- Dramatically reduced amount of inflammation

- Increased feeling of well-being due to reduction of inflammation

Gundry also recommends, in addition, a herbal laxative. However, I do not find this necessary. If you follow the recommendations, this should be enough to cleanse the intestines.

PHASE 2: REPAIR AND RESTORE

The first phase accomplished, well done! Now you are ready for the more enjoyable part, namely choosing from a much larger list of foods.

Now it is up to you to stay focused on the plan for another six weeks and only to consume foods from the positive list. This way, the intestines can regenerate and get ready for the new type of nutrition. Inflamed tissue in the gut can heal and come to rest. The intestinal flora will be fortified in a positive way.

Please note that you should not eat more than 120 grams of animal protein per meal.

Vegetarians and vegans can refer to the vegetarian and vegan recipes included here or simply replace the animal proteins with Tempeh, hemp tofu, vegan eggs, pressure-cooked legumes or cauliflower "steaks". Acceptable Quorn products are also an alternative.

Warning: According to Dr. Gundry, in this phase it is possible to suffer withdrawal symptoms, in the form of headaches, muscle cramps or loss of energy. He explains this as a dependence of our bodies on all these foods, which we eat daily and which make us sick: Grain, in particular whole wheat, specific vegetable and fruit types, sugar etc.

This phase is mainly aimed at introducing you to new dishes. I experimented a lot during this phase with cabbage varieties which I had previously not integrated much into my diet. Today, I cannot think of being without them. I did not suffer from the type of withdrawal symptoms which Gundry describes. This does not mean that it will not affect you. It is important to note that everybody reacts differently.

RULES DURING PHASE 2:

Gundry recommends adhering to the following rules during Phase 2:

- All foods which contain appreciable amounts of Lectins, plant pesticides, GMO (genetically manipulated organisms) etc. should be avoided.

- All sugar and artificial sweeteners should also be avoided.

- Avoid also Omega 6 fats.

- Do not eat any more poultry or fish from industrial farming, or milk products from cattle reared by intensive mass animal farming, which have been fed with antibiotics, corn, soy etc.

- Very small amounts of nuts or avocado are allowed

- All hormone-disrupting products (i.e. personal care products, deodorants, plastic etc) are forbidden.

The following may be consumed:

- All types of greens (lettuces), tubers and root vegetables and resistant starches.

- More Omega 3 fats from fish, lentils and possibly MCT oil.

- No more than max. 120 grams of meat per day (incl. fish)

- Milk products only from A2 cows, sheep, buffalo or goats

PHASE 3: REAP THE REWARDS

After those six weeks you will be more familiar with the food lists. Your body has begun to regenerate. Do you notice the change? Do you have less stomach ache and a feeling of increased well-being?

Not everyone regenerates at the same pace. Some notice the recovery of their intestinal flora already after 4 weeks and for others it can take longer than 6 weeks. This is different for each individual and cannot be influenced.

Take notice of your body's signals. If you have the feeling that your intestines are improving and you are suffering from fewer symptoms, you can begin Phase 3 and attempt to consume Lectin richer foods. The focus continues to lie on the consumption of positive foods. If you sometimes take foods from the negative list, notice how your body reacts to it. Begin with small amounts.

In the 3rd phase, you should reduce consumption of animal proteins (including fish) to between 60 and 120 grams per day.

This phase has no time limit. I regard it as my new way of eating. This phase could become your companion for the future.

INTERMITTENT FASTING

For those of us who live in industrial countries, it is normal to have access to a continual supply of food. After all, we have a surplus of food.

Our ancestors, who were hunters and gatherers, did not have that surplus. Before humans became settled and learned to become crop and animal farmers, there were always days when they did not have food available and they had to fast.

This seems quite dramatic to our pampered ears, but this involuntary fasting in no way damaged us. On the contrary, it unburdened our organisms and made us more resilient.

You can integrate intermittent fasting into Phase 3 in order to strengthen your organisms. There are several ways to do this. You can, for example fast on one or two days a week. You decide yourself how long to fast for. The more hours you fast, the greater the effect.

I personally find it easiest to skip breakfast and eat my first meal at 11 or 12 o'clock. After that I would eat a snack and have dinner at 5 or 6 o'clock in the evening. This way I can fast for 16 to 18 hours, depending on how I organise it. I try to do that 2 or 3 times a week, depending on my schedule. I only drink water during fasting times and not too much, only enough to quench the thirst.

THE KETO INTENSIVE CARE PROGRAMME

Nutrition in the ketogenic diet is based on the principle: Fewer carbohydrates, fewer proteins but a lot of fat. Normally, the body draws its energy from carbohydrates. If this energy source is not available, the metabolism changes into a ketogenic state.

In the liver, fats are transformed into so-called ketones. These are used to obtain energy instead of the carbohydrates in order to maintain, for example, the performance of your brain. This condition is called "ketosis" and is the principle on which the ketogenic diet relies.

Gundry developed a nutritional concept for exactly that purpose. In this book I do not want to expand more on this type of nutrition. Instead I would like to focus on the 3 phases involved in achieving a low-Lectin diet.

Nevertheless, you can find markings, on the positive food list, which identify the foods used in the keto-intensive programme. This can be useful if you want to follow this subject more closely and also serves to provide a more complete list of foods.

OTHER DISRUPTIVE FACTORS WHICH DISABLE A HEALTHY GUT

Gundry names similar disruptive factors for the gut as previously mentioned under Leaky Gut Syndrome. It is prudent to avoid these in order to maintain healthy intestinal flora.

BROAD SPECTRUM ANTIBIOTICS

Broad spectrum antibiotics kill nearly all bacteria, good and bad. This type of antibiotic should only be taken in the worst of emergencies. Unfortunately, these antibiotics are often used in livestock farming in order to prevent diseases in animals, particularly in intensive livestock farming. In this way, it (and other dangerous substances) arrive in meat products, then indirectly, by eating the meat, into humans. For this reason, Gundry recommends avoiding consumption of all meat products unless they are traditionally raised, grass-fed and have not received medicines, such as antibiotics.

NON-STEROIDAL ANTI-INFLAMMATORY DRUGS (NSAIDS)

The painkiller group of non-steroidal anti-inflammatory drugs, such as Aspirin, Ibuprofen etc., affect strongly the intestinal wall and can cause permanent damage.

GASTRIC ACID BLOCKING AGENTS (PROTON PUMP INHIBITORS, PPI)

According to Gundry, these should be avoided under any circumstances because they reduce the amount of gastric acid in the body which can lead to a shut down in large sections of the immune system. Bacteria which is damaging for us is no longer eliminated by the acid and can cause great damage to the microbiomes in the intestines.

Today, this group of medicines is often prescribed as a "stomach protection". A gastric acid blocking agent is often prescribed, particularly for those patients who have to take a lot of medication, so that the stomach lining can be protected. In conventional medicine, these blockers are considered to be unproblematic with very few side effects. Because of this, they are often prescribed after the principle: "Even if it does not work, it will not harm". Gundry does not believe that this is the case, if you take into consideration their effect on the intestines.

ARTIFICIAL SWEETENERS

This substance group also has a strong influence on our intestinal flora, according to Gundry. These substances activate a "fat storage mode" in our bodies, independent of whether they are "real" sugar or sweeteners. It is the sweetness which, Gundry says, is the signal. The only safe sweeteners are: Stevia, Xylitol, Erythritol and Inulin.

HORMONE SYSTEM DISRUPTORS

These are all substances and substance groups which work like oestrogens. These can be found in almost all plastics (BPA/Phthalates), cash register receipts, dichlorodifenyl-dichloroethylene (DDE), polychlorinated biphenyl (PCB), preservatives (including Parabens). All cause "devastation" in our hormone systems leading to multiple problems:

- Overweight, diabetes and other metabolic diseases

- Dysfunctions in reproductive organs (men and women)

- Cancers in women, who have had hormone problems

- Problems with prostate gland

- Problems with thyroid glands

- Problems in brain development and neuro-endocrine systems.

- Vitamin D reserve exhausted (reduction of the liver function needed to convert this vitamin into its active form)

- Oestrogen dominance leading to male breasts and fat accumulation.

GENETIC MODIFIED ORGANISMS (GMO):

Here, proteins, including Lectins are introduced into plants, which are intended to protect against insects. As a result, we consume these proteins from the genetically modified plants in our food. Farming genetically modified plants often leads to an increased use in herbicides. The most common of these includes the active ingredient Glyphosate, and the herbicide is known as Roundup. Genetically modified plants also produce their own insecticide. These substances are an added risk to our health.

BLUE LIGHT:

Our circadian rhythm is guided by blue light which, among other things, influences our Melatonin production (our sleep-wake rhythm), Ghrelin (appetite) and Cortisol (stress hormone). The blue light from OLED and LCD displays from TVs, computers, smart phones and cold light (LED and energy-saving bulbs) causes our biorhythm to become completely confused. The body recognises it as being always day and always Summer which, according to Gundry, means for the body: Fat storage!

LOSING WEIGHT WITHOUT LECTINS

When considering diets and the wish to lose weight, it is worth taking a look at Lectins. These days, there are so many diets and all claim to be the most helpful to let the weight fall off. Some really do help to lose weight in the short term. However, how do you keep off the weight once you have lost it?

WHY LOW-CARB DIETS DO NOT HELP LONG-TERM

During a low-carb diet, carbohydrates are greatly reduced. These days, this diet form is very popular and many think it is the key to losing weight. Even Gundry successfully lost weight, using a low-carb diet, unfortunately without a positive long-term outcome. And here lies the problem. Avoiding carbohydrates does have a short-term positive effect – you lose weight. However, when you start again to eat food with Lectin-containing carbohydrates (from grain, corns and seeds), the pounds return quickly.

Carbohydrate consumption is drastically reduced in all low-carb diets. The foods containing grain and legumes are avoided and with it, much of the Lectins. This has a positive effect on the body. Subsequently, if you eat wholemeal bread, pasta and legumes once again after the diet, it causes a yoyo effect. Gundry's recommendation: Stay away from grains and legumes (Lectins).

THE PALEO CONCEPT

The Paleo diet is also called the Stone Age diet. This also involves the consumption of very few carbohydrates but uses a lot of protein. The concept of the Paleo diet is based on the consumption of Stone Age people as we assume, that they ate only a little in the way of carbohydrates. A lot of protein was consumed by eating the meat from buffalos, mammoths and antelopes (also their fat). However, the weight loss and improvement in health achieved during the paleo or another low-carb diet is not due to the avoidance of carbohydrates and the consumption of high-protein fish, meat and fat. The positive effects were more likely to have been caused by the reduction in carbohydrates resulting in the minimisation of Lectin consumption. It is important to note with the Paleo diet, Stone Age animals were surely not fed with grains, corn or soy products. This means, that the meat contained no Lectins in contrast to our meat of today (except in specifically grain- corn- or soy-free fed animals).

The geographical area also plays a role. In Africa, where our ancestors of 100,000 years ago came from, there were absolutely no Lectin-containing plants or vegetables. All the Lectin-containing food of today, such as tomatoes, cucumbers, courgettes, peppers, cashew nuts, sunflower seeds, pumpkin seeds and Chia seeds, originate from the transatlantic world and should not be consumed in a low-Lectin diet.

THE KETO DIET

The Ketogenic diet is usually recommended, or even prescribed, for people (also children) who suffer from diabetes in order to reduce their blood glucose and insulin levels.

The Ketogenic diet is also a version of the low carbohydrate diet, although there is a significant difference: Instead of consuming more proteins, as in the Paleo diet, the real Ketogenic diet also limits protein. Keto is low-carbohydrate and high fat. The Keto concept: No fear of fat!

Because this diet recommends the reduction of carbohydrates, the Lectins are also automatically reduced and accordingly there is an automatic weight-loss. If this is combined with a Keto diet variant, it can even produce positive results, not only in diabetes patients who are extremely resistant to insulin, but also in patients with arterial sclerosis, cancer, dementia, Parkinson's, MS, autoimmune diseases and diseases of the intestinal tract.

RECIPES

BREAKFAST

CRUNCHY MUESLI

Phases 2-3
Portion: for 200 g muesli mix
Preparation time: 5 minutes plus 10 minutes cooking time.

Ingredients:
- Millet flakes
- Linseed
- Coconut flakes
- Sesame
- Chopped and flaked almonds
- Birch sugar
- Coconut oil
- Dried dates / figs
- Goat yoghurt

Pre-heat the oven to 150°C

Warm the coconut oil and mix with the birch sugar. Pour over the muesli mix. Mix well.

Lay the pre-steeped and still moist grain mix onto a baking tray and press well. Bake for approximately 10 minutes. Check regularly that the mix does not brown too much.

Let the mix cool overnight and subsequently break into small pieces.

Note that coconut oil turns liquid at a temperature of 25°C, so it is preferable to store the crunchy muesli in the fridge.

As a variation, you can cut two dried dates or an unsweetened fig into small pieces and add them to the muesli. You can also add a small beaker of goat yoghurt or almond milk. There are no limits to your (lectin-free) fantasy in this respect. Walnuts or hazelnuts taste wonderful in the muesli and make it crunchier. Or you can add Psyllium husks, pistachios, pecan nuts, hemp seeds or chestnut flakes as you wish. The latter are not so easily available.

SUNDAY BREAD BUNS

Phases 2 -3

Portions: 1

Total preparation time: 10 minutes plus 15 minutes baking time

Ingredients:

- 180g ground almonds
- 2 tablespoonfuls desiccated coconut
- 30g Linseed meal
- 2 tablespoonfuls cream of tartar baking powder (natural alternative to conventional baking powder)
- 5 eggs (organic and from the meadow or pasture)
- 40g coconut oil
- 1 pinch of salt
- 1 tablespoonfuls apple vinegar
- Sesame or linseed for decoration.

Preheat the oven to 180°C. Place the ground almonds, desiccated coconut, linseed meal, baking powder and salt in a large bowl. Melt the coconut oil and mix with the eggs and apple vinegar. Form it into 6 small bread buns (moisten the hands to avoid the dough sticking to them). Sprinkle the sesame or linseed over the top.

Bake for 15 minutes.

Tip: The bread buns are suitable for freezing. If you make them slightly flatter, you can thaw them by putting them in the toaster. They taste at least as good as the non-frozen ones, if not better, because they are a little crispier.

SMOOTHIES

GREEN SMOOTHIE

Phases 1-3
Portion: 1
Total preparation time: 5 minutes

Ingredients:
- 1 cup of chopped Romaine lettuce
- 1/2 cup baby spinach
- 1 sprig of mint with stem
- 1/2 avocado
- 4 tablespoonfuls freshly squeezed lemon juice
- 3 – 6 drops Stevia-extract
- ¼ cup ice cubes
- 1 cup water

Put all ingredients into a smoothie maker and blend them until the mixture is smooth and fluffy. Add more ice cubes as desired.

If the smoothie is too thick, you can add a little water to it. It is also possible to make three portions and place the rest into the fridge for a maximum of 3 days in a closed receptacle. This is particularly recommended during Phase 1 as you will be consuming the smoothie for three days for breakfast.

Instead of Stevia you can add more mint and lemon juice.

AVOCADO FIG SMOOTHIE

Phases 2-3

Portions: 1

Total preparation time: 5 minutes

Ingredients:
- 1 half avocado
- 1 handful kale
- 1 sprig mint
- Pulp from 1 orange
- 2 dried figs
- Juice of half lemon
- 1 cup water
- ¼ cup ice cubes

Place all ingredients in a smoothie maker and blend them until the mixture is smooth and fluffy. Add more ice cubes as desired. If the smoothie is too thick, add a little water.

SNACKS

CABBAGE CRISPS

Phases 1-3
Portions: 2
Total preparation time: 10 minutes plus 30-40 minutes baking time

Ingredients:
- about 3 savoy cabbage leaves
- 3 tablespoonfuls olive oil
- 1 teaspoonful sea salt

Pre-heat the oven to 130°C. Tear the savoy cabbage leaves into pieces of about 5 x 5 cm, not too small, the cabbage crisps shrink a little in the oven.

Place some baking paper onto a baking tray and spread the cabbage pieces onto it.

Mix the olive oil and sea salt in a small bowl and spread the mixture evenly onto the cabbage with a brush. Do not put too much oil onto the cabbage so that it stays crispy.

Bake for about 30 – 40 minutes. Check regularly that the crisps do not get too dark.

COCONUT YOGHURT WITH DRIED FRUIT

Phases 2 – 3

Portions: 1

Total preparation time: 5 minutes.

Ingredients:
- Coconut yoghurt – about 100g per person.
- Dried apricots
- Raisins
- Chopped almonds
- Cocoa nibs
- Maple syrup for the vegan variation or, if preferred, honey to sweeten.

Chop the dried fruits finely and mix them with the almonds and cocoa nibs. Fold into the coconut yoghurt.

Sweeten as preferred with honey or syrup. I always do this right at the end as the sweetness from the fruits is sometimes enough and I need less than I thought.

At the end, lay a few pieces of fruit on the top and you are finished.

You can add other types of fruit as you wish. This makes a tasty breakfast or dessert.

ROMAINE LETTUCE BOATS FILLED WITH GUACAMOLE

Phases 1 – 3

Portions: 1

Total preparation time: 5 minutes

Ingredients:

- ½ avocado
- 1 tablespoonfuls finely chopped red onion
- 1 teaspoonful finely chopped coriander
- 1 tablespoonful freshly squeezed lemon juice
- 1 pinch of sea salt, preferably iodised
- 4 leaves Romaine lettuce, washed and patted dry.

Mix the avocado with the lemon juice and season with a little salt. Blend them together with the onion and coriander until the mixture is smooth. Add the mixture to the romaine lettuce leaves.

MAIN COURSES

ASIA WRAP WITH CHICKEN AND CORIANDER DIP

Phases 1 – 3
Portions: 1
Total preparation time: 15 minutes

Ingredients:

Filling
- 1 tablespoonful avocado oil
- 120g chicken breast without skin, cut in 1cm thick strips
- 2 tablespoonfuls freshly squeezed lemon juice
- ¼ teaspoonful sea salt, preferably iodised, plus extra to taste
- ½ avocado, cut in cubes
- 1 cup rocket
- 1 leaf Nori (Sushi algae)
- 4 green olives, stoned and halved

Coriander Dip
- 2 cups chopped coriander
- ¼ cup native olive oil extra

- 2 tablespoonfuls freshly squeezed lemon juice
- ¼ teaspoon sea salt, preferably iodised.

Nori is a form of seaweed, which has been flattened into squares or strips. This is an excellent substitute for flatbread. A bamboo mat, such as those found in the Asian section of the majority of supermarkets, can help you to form tight seaweed rolls.

For the filling add the avocado oil into a small pan and heat on a high setting. Add the chicken strips and 1 tablespoonful lemon juice and salt. Fry the chicken strips for about 2 minutes each side or until cooked through. Add the avocado and the rest of the lemon juice and season with salt.

For the dip, place all ingredients in a powerful mixer and blend.

Lay the rocket onto the lower half of the seaweed sheets and place the chicken on top. Add the avocado and olives. Sprinkle with salt. Roll carefully into tight rolls and close the ends with a little water. Cut into halves and serve with the coriander dip.

Vegan version: Substitute the chicken with corn-free Tempeh, hemp tofu or a cauliflower "steak" (a 1cm thick slice of cauliflower, fried at a high temperature in avocado oil).

Vegetarian version: As above, or substitute with an acceptable Quorn product.

Avocado oil can be substituted with olive oil or sesame oil as preferred.

ROASTED BROCCOLI WITH CAULIFLOWER RICE AND SAUTÉED ONIONS

Phases 1 – 3

Portions: 1

Total preparation time: 20 minutes

Ingredients:

<u>Cauliflower rice:</u>
- ½ head of a mid-sized cauliflower
- 1 tablespoonful avocado oil
- 1 tablespoonful freshly squeezed lemon juice
- ¼ teaspoonful curry powder
- 1 pinch of sea salt, preferably iodised

<u>Broccoli:</u>
- 1 ½ cups chopped broccoli
- 1 ½ tablespoonfuls avocado oil
- 1 pinch of sea salt, preferably iodised

<u>Onions:</u>
- 1 onion
- ½ tablespoonful avocado oil
- 1 pinch sea salt, preferably iodised

To prepare the cauliflower rice, grate the cauliflower with the largest section of the cheese grater into rice-like pieces. You can also serve this rice with other main dishes.

Heat the oven to 160°C.

Place the cauliflower into a medium-sized frying pan together with a tablespoonful of avocado oil, lemon juice, curry powder and a pinch of salt. Fry for 3 to 5 minutes. Take care not to fry for too long, or the mixture will turn mushy. Take the cauliflower rice out of the pan and keep warm on a plate.

Wipe the pan with a paper towel.

Put the broccoli in an oven dish and add one tablespoonful avocado oil. Roast for 15 minutes or until the broccoli is soft, stirring twice during that time. Season with a pinch of salt.

Heat the rest of the avocado oil in the frying pan at a medium setting. Add the onions, which have been cut into slices and fry them until they are crispy. Season with a pinch of salt.

Serve the cauliflower rice on a plate and spread the broccoli and fried onions over it.

The avocado oil can be substituted with olive oil or sesame oil as preferred.

CABBAGE KALE SAUTÉE WITH SALMON AND AVOCADO

Phases 1 – 3
Portions: 1
Total preparation time: 20 minutes

This recipe is very flexible. You can substitute the salmon for another wild-caught fish, shellfish or chicken. You can use Bok Choy or Napa cabbage (also known as celery cabbage) instead of kale.

Ingredients:

- ½ avocado cut into cubes
- 3 tablespoonfuls freshly squeezed lemon juice
- 4 pinches of sea salt, preferably iodised
- 3 tablespoonfuls avocado oil
- 1 ½ cups finely chopped kale
- ½ red onion, cut thinly
- 100g wild-caught Alaska salmon

Sprinkle the cubed avocado pieces with 1 tablespoonful lemon juice and season with a pinch of salt. Set the avocados to the side. Warm a frying pan on a medium heat setting and, as soon as it is warm, add 2 tablespoonfuls avocado oil, the kale and the onions. Fry for about 10 minutes until tender, stirring occasionally. Season with a further two pinches of salt. Remove from the pan and set aside.

Add one tablespoonful avocado oil into the pan. Increase the heat, add the rest of the lemon juice and the salmon. Fry the salmon until cooked, turning after 3 minutes (a total of about 6 minutes). Season with a pinch of salt. Serve with the sautéed kale and the onions and garnish with avocado.

Vegan version: Substitute the chicken with corn-free Tempeh, hemp tofu or a cauliflower "steak": A 1cm thick slice of cauliflower fried in hot avocado oil.

Vegetarian version: As above or substitute with an acceptable Quorn product.

The avocado oil can be substituted with olive oil of sesame oil as preferred.

LENTIL SALAD WITH SESAME DRESSING

Phases 2 – 3

Portions: 1

Total preparation time: 10 minutes plus 30 minutes cooking time for the lentils.

Ingredients:

For the lentil salad:
- 1 cup Beluga lentils
- 2 carrots
- 2 spring onions
- 1 large handful rocket
- 3 full sprigs of mint
- 1 handful coriander
- Sesame grains to garnish.

For the dressing:
- 3 tablespoonfuls sesame tahini (sesame cream)
- 4 tablespoonfuls olive oil
- 4 tablespoonfuls lemon juice or vinegar (e.g. apple vinegar)
- 1 tablespoonful mustard
- 2 tablespoonfuls water

- Salt and pepper

Boil the lentils. Beluga lentils need a cooking time of at least 30 minutes. Take care that the lentils are still firm to the bite. Allow the lentils to cool a little.

In the meantime, peel the carrots and cut them into rough pieces. Cook them in boiling water for about 5 minutes until they are soft, but still firm to the bite. Coarsely grate the carrots.

Wash the spring onion, rocket, mint and coriander and chop coarsely.

Add all the fresh ingredients to the cooled lentils.

For the sesame dressing mix all ingredients, apart from the oil, in a bowl and mix them with a whisk or fork. Add the olive oil, little by little. This is important to avoid the mix from curdling. Add salt and pepper to taste. If you have a large number of lentils, you can stretch the dressing with a little water.

Pour the dressing over the salad and mix well. The lentil salad tastes best with sesame dressing if it is allowed to steep for a few hours.

Finally, add a few sesame grains over the top, this gives it a bit of bite.

ROMAINE SALAD WITH AVOCADO AND BASIL PESTO CHICKEN

Phases: 1 – 3

Portions: 1

Total preparation time: 15 minutes

Ingredients:

<u>Chicken:</u>
- 1 tablespoonful avocado oil
- 120g chicken breast without skin cut into 1cm thick strips
- 1 tablespoonful freshly squeezed lemon juice
- ¼ teaspoonful sea salt, preferably iodised

<u>Pesto:</u>
- 2 cups chopped basil
- ¼ cup native olive oil extra
- 2 tablespoonfuls freshly squeezed lemon juice
- ¼ teaspoonful salt, preferably iodised

<u>Dressing:</u>
- ½ avocado, cut into cubes

- 2 tablespoonfuls freshly squeezed lemon juice
- 2 tablespoonfuls native olive oil extra
- 1 pinch of sea salt, preferably iodised

Salad:

- 1 ½ cups chopped romaine lettuce
- Chopped radish (optional)

Heat the avocado oil in a small frying pan on a hot setting. Add the chicken strips and sprinkle with lemon juice and salt. Fry the chicken strips for 2 minutes on each side or until they are cooked through.

For the pesto, place all ingredients into a powerful mixer and blend them.

Sprinkle the avocado cubes with 1 tablespoonful lemon juice and season with a pinch of salt. Put the remaining lemon juice, olive oil and salt into a preserving jar with a tight-fitting lid and shake until all the ingredients are well mixed.

Put the romaine lettuce and dressing into deep plate. Lay the avocado and chicken onto the salad and spread the pesto over the top.

Vegan version: Substitute the chicken with corn-free Tempeh, hemp tofu or a cauliflower "steak": A 1cm thick slice of cauliflower fried in hot avocado oil.

Vegetarian version: As above or substitute with an acceptable Quorn product.

The avocado oil can be substituted with olive oil of sesame oil as preferred.

You can substitute the basil with coriander or parsley, whichever taste you prefer.

ROCKET SALAD WITH CHICKEN AND LEMON VINAIGRETTE

Phases 1 – 3

Portions: 1

Total preparation time: 15 minutes

Ingredients:

Chicken:

- 1 tablespoonful avocado oil
- 120g chicken breast cut into 1cm thick strips
- 1 tablespoonful freshly squeezed lemon juice
- ¼ teaspoonful sea salt, preferably iodised
- ½ lemon peel (optional)

Dressing:

- 2 tablespoonfuls native olive oil extra
- 1 tablespoonful freshly squeezed lemon juice
- 1 pinch sea salt, preferably iodised

Salad:

- 1 ½ cups rocket

Heat the avocado oil in a small frying pan on a hot setting. Add the chicken strips and sprinkle with lemon juice and salt. Fry the chicken strips on both sides for 2 minutes each or until they are fully cooked.

For the dressing you can put the ingredients in a preserving jar with a tightly-fitting lid. Shake well until all the ingredients are mixed.

Fold the rocket into the dressing and garnish with the chicken. Add the lemon peel if desired.

Vegan version: Substitute the chicken with corn-free Tempeh, hemp tofu or a cauliflower "steak": A 1cm thick slice of cauliflower fried in hot avocado oil.

Vegetarian version: As above or substitute with an acceptable Quorn product.

The avocado oil can be substituted with olive oil of sesame oil as preferred.

LEMONY BRUSSEL SPROUTS, KALE AND ONIONS WITH CABBAGE STEAK

Phases 1 – 3
Portions 1
Total preparation time: 20 minutes

Ingredients:

- 4 tablespoonfuls avocado oil
- A 2.5cm thick slice of red cabbage
- ¼ teaspoonful plus 1 pinch sea salt, preferably iodised
- ½ red onion, cut thinly
- 1 cup sprouts, cut thinly
- 1 ½ cups kale, chopped
- 1 tablespoonful freshly squeezed lemon juice
- Olive oil extra virgin (optional)

Heat one tablespoonful of avocado oil in a frying pan. Reduce heat to medium setting and fry the red cabbage slice until it is golden brown on both sides, about 3 minutes on each side. Season with a pinch of salt. Place on a plate and keep warm.

Heat 2 tablespoonfuls avocado oil in the frying pan at a medium setting. Add the onion and sprouts. Fry them until they are tender, about 3 minutes.

Add 1 tablespoonful avocado oil, the kale and the lemon juice and fry everything for a further 3 minutes. Season with salt.

Serve the cabbage steak, topped with the fried vegetables. Add olive oil if desired.

The avocado oil can be substituted with olive oil of sesame oil as preferred.

Use one of the many types of cabbage for this recipe. If you do not use kale, make sure to remove the thick stalks before chopping. If you are using kale, you can chop the stalks in with it.

CONCLUSION

The plant world is very clever about how it can protect the so-called Lectins against its enemies using certain substances. Unfortunately, these have a negative impact on our bodies. That set me to thinking and I asked myself: Does it really have to be, that we eat plants every day, containing substances which damage our bodies? Is it not so, that plants are really protecting themselves from humans and give us signals that we should leave them alone?

Looking more closely, I saw, that the negative impact is greater than the positive one. In fact, we run the danger of developing diseases.

By consuming high-Lectin foods, the risk of developing autoimmune diseases grows.

High-Lectin food, which we like to eat these days, could be the reason that we so often suffer from autoimmune diseases, allergies and other ailments.

One fact which I find shocking, is that Lectins could be responsible for the leaky gut syndrome, which has become an important factor for me. Even if you do not suffer from that, I think it is enormously important that you understand the link between the leaky gut syndrome and Lectins. This does not mean that holes are already present but that, if you continue to eat high-lectin foods, you greatly increase the risk to find holes in your intestines.

It is a shame that traditional medicine has not yet shown much interest in the leaky gut syndrome. Perhaps it is the key to the treatment of many autoimmune diseases. If you take that thought a step further, you could suppose that traditional medicine does not want to follow that lead, because the medicinal treatment, and with it the profit margins in the health care sector, would sink. This may not be the case. It is much more probable that traditional medicine is simply focusing on student-based research. There is probably more study and research required to establish the links between Lectins, leaky gut syndrome and autoimmune diseases. If such a link were found, it would probably be given a lot more importance.

I find Gundry's theory and his nutritional concept a very helpful programme to enable a change in diet, leading to weight loss and a reduction in long-term disorders. He is a pioneer in this field and he relies on his own findings gained from his patients. His views are sometimes criticised by supporters of other types of nutrition. I believe that this is a very interesting and logical concept. Every concept has its origins somewhere, where people have made significant discoveries based on their own experiences and knowledge. I hope that there will be more research in this area and that Gundry's theory will appeal to a growing number of people.

Through my own experience, I recommend the change in diet to all those who would like to pursue a healthy nutritional scheme, which can positively influence the gut and body, at the same time helping them to lose weight and keep the weight off.

My stomach aches, which originated from damaged intestinal flora, have almost completely disappeared, due to the change in diet. After about the first month and in the second phase, I noticed a significant improvement in my digestion and that has remained to this day.

I still eat mostly low-Lectin foods, although I do eat some food with Lectins, but consciously, not often and in small amounts. I try to carry out the intermittent fasting 2 to 3 times per week by not eating breakfast, thereby increasing the length of time between the evening meal and the next meal, in order to give my intestines time to complete the digestive process. I find that surprisingly easy to do, particularly as I was never a big breakfast-eater.

The most difficult part of this type of diet is when you want to eat out. In the meantime, I invite friends and family mostly to my home to eat or we cook together. I noticed that people who are not familiar with this type of eating are quickly out of their depth. I can make exceptions if I eat only small amounts of high-Lectin food. In restaurants I weigh up which foods have the least Lectins and that is how I choose what I will eat. For example, I sometimes ask if I can have a low-Lectin substitute for a particular type of vegetable.

In the preparation, I pay attention to the recommended cooking variation. The germination of Lectins is often described in literature. Gundry does not give much importance to the germination process.

He believes you cannot really reduce the Lectins much in this respect. As it is not clear how useful germination is, I prefer other cooking variations. For example, I often use my steam pressure cooker and I recommend highly purchasing one. It is really practical and enables me to reduce Lectins to the minimum.

Most important for me is the correct form of nutrition, despite having to deal with various restrictions in everyday life. I am glad to have found this subject and to have come to terms with it. Now I have my symptoms under control and generally feel healthier, most probably because of my healthy gut.

I recommend giving a low-Lectin diet a chance and to see how it benefits you. Do you feel better? Are the symptoms better under control? If yes, stick with it. The long-term change in diet is the key to improvement in your health. I wish you much success with it.

DID YOU ENJOY MY BOOK?

Now you have read my book, you know to use permaculture to make the world a better place. This is why I am asking you now for a small favour. Customer reviews are an important part of every product offered by Amazon. It is the first thing that customers look at and, more often than not, is the main reason whether or not they decide to buy the product. Considering the endless number of products available at Amazon, this factor is becoming increasingly important.

If you liked my book, I would be more than grateful if you could leave your review by Amazon. How do you do that? Just click on the "Write a customer review"-button (as shown below), which you find on the Amazon product page of my book or your orders site:

Review this product

Share your thoughts with other customers

Write a customer review

Please write a short note explaining what you liked most and what you found to be most important. It will not take longer than a few minutes, promise!

Be assured, I will read every review personally. It will help me a lot to improve my books and to tailor them to your wishes.

For this I say to you:

Thank you very much!

Yours
Lutz

REFERENCES

The Plant Paradox: The Hidden Dangers in "Healthy" Foods That Cause Disease and Weight Gain, Steven R. Gundry, 25. April 2017

Lectins and glycobiology, hrsg. von Gabius, Hans-Joachim [¬Hrsg.], 1993

Plant lectins, von Pusztai, Arpad, 1991

Systematik des Pflanzenreichs: unter besonderer Berücksichtigung chemischer Merkmale und pflanzlicher Drogen, von Frohne, Dietrich, 1998

Lectins, 2 ed., von H. Lis Nathan Sharon, 2007

Lectins: biomedical perspectives, von Bardocz, Susan Pusztai, Arpad, 21.04.2014

Böses Gemüse: Wie gesunde Nahrungsmittel uns krank machen. Lektine - die versteckte Gefahr im Essen, Steven R. Gundry, 07. Februar 2018

https://autoimmunportal.de/leaky-gut-syndrom/

https://reizdarm.one/ernaehrung/lektine/

https://www.lebensmittellexikon.de/

https://german.mercola.com/sites/articles/archive/2018/04/19/reduzierung-von-lektinen-in-der-ernahrung.aspx

https://www.mdr.de/wissen/mensch-alltag/boeses-gemuese-100.html

https://www.4blutgruppen.de/lektine/

https://www.privatkoch-hamburg.de/fermentiertes-gemuese/

https://www.milch.info/milchsorten/a2-milch/

https://www.ncbi.nlm.nih.gov/pubmed/10884708?dopt=AbstractPlus

https://humanfoodbar.com/plant-paradox-recipes/

http://www.leafygreens.de/category/rezepte/

BOOK RECOMMENDATIONS

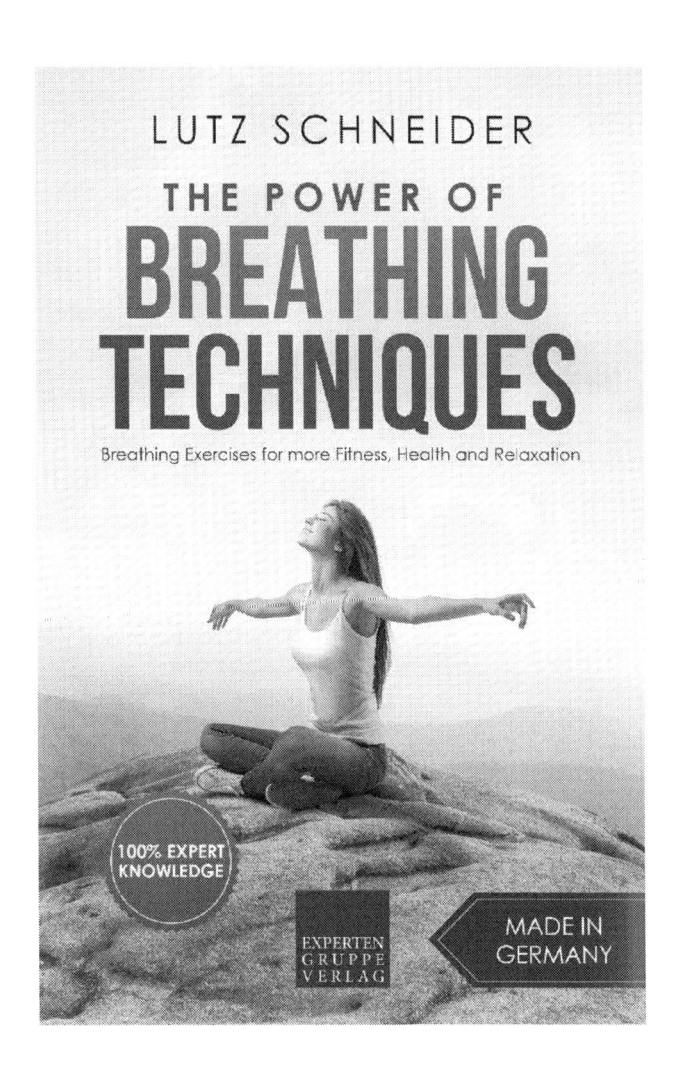

The Power of Breathing Techniques

Breathing Exercises for more Fitness, Health and Relaxation

We can survive for weeks without food and days without water, but only a few minutes without air.

Would it not be justified to presume that the air, which is more important for human survival than food or water, should live up to basic standards? How much air do we need for ideal breathing? And how should we breathe?

The amount of air that you breathe has the potential to change everything you believe about your body, your health and your performance.

In this book, you will discover the fundamental relationship between Oxygen and your body.

Increasing your Oxygen supply is not only healthy, it enables an increase in the intensity of your training and also reduces breathlessness. In short, you will notice an improvement in your health and more relaxation in your everyday life.

Look forward to reading a lot of background information, experience reports, step-by-step instructions and secret tips which are tailor-made to your breathing technique and help you to become fitter, healthier and more relaxed.

This book is available on Amazon!

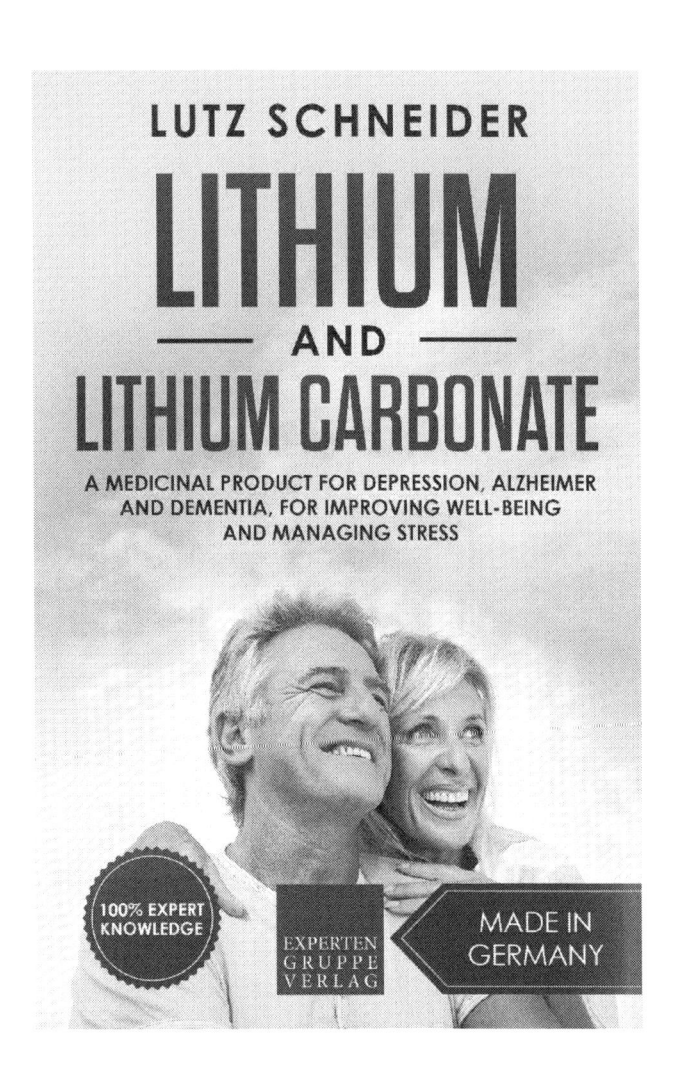

LUTZ SCHNEIDER
LITHIUM
— AND —
LITHIUM CARBONATE

A MEDICINAL PRODUCT FOR DEPRESSION, ALZHEIMER AND DEMENTIA, FOR IMPROVING WELL-BEING AND MANAGING STRESS

100% EXPERT KNOWLEDGE

EXPERTEN GRUPPE VERLAG

MADE IN GERMANY

Lithium and Lithium Carbonate

A medicinal product for Depression, Alzheimer and Dementia, for improving well-being and managing stress

Lithium is mostly known for its use in batteries. Most people do not realise that it is also a trace element in our bodies.

Would it not be wonderful if you could fight sicknesses, such as depression or Alzheimer, and improve your well-being, if you just had a little more Lithium in your body? What if you did not have to do anything more than take a little more Lithium?

Lithium is an important component for all of us in achieving a lasting, healthy way of life. Clinical studies and scientific articles are speaking a clear language. Despite that, Lithium is suffering a niche existence by a large majority of pharmaceutical scientists and is hardly known by the broad population.

Even so, the advantages of Lithium, which lie in psychological and mental health sector, are obvious and it is easy to obtain and use.

In this book, you will discover the advantages and effects of Lithium on your body and mind.

Read about fascinating background information, scientific findings, experience reports and secret tips which are tailor-made for your needs and which will help you to achieve a healthy, longer and more fulfilling life.

This book is available on Amazon!

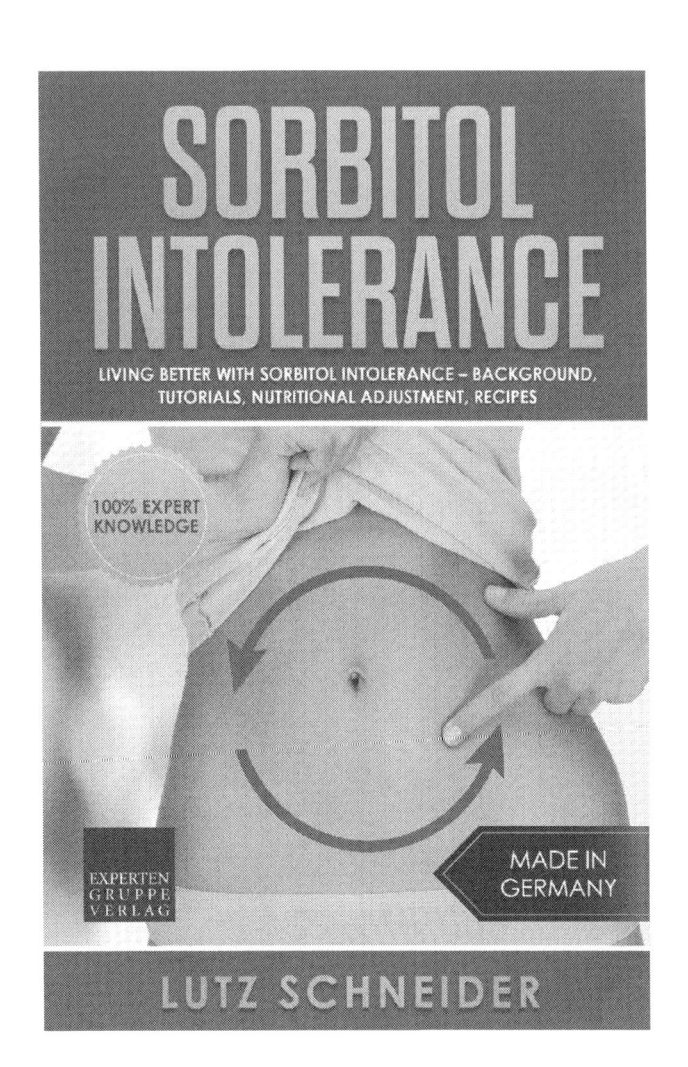

SORBITOL INTOLERANCE

LIVING BETTER WITH SORBITOL INTOLERANCE – BACKGROUND, TUTORIALS, NUTRITIONAL ADJUSTMENT, RECIPES

100% EXPERT KNOWLEDGE

EXPERTEN GRUPPE VERLAG

MADE IN GERMANY

LUTZ SCHNEIDER

Sorbitol Intolerance

Living better with Sorbitol intolerance – background, tutorials, nutritional adjustment, recipes

Sorbitol intolerance is one of the least known food intolerances among many. And that, even though more and more people are suffering from it.

Wouldn't it be wonderful if you could at last find out if you suffer from Sorbitol intolerance? And how can you eat a diverse and delicious diet, despite your Sorbitol intolerance?

An increasing amount of industrially prepared food means that more and more people are taking doses of Sorbitol which they are not able to digest properly. This leads to a large number of lingering symptoms which are difficult to assign to any particular substance.

In this book you will find a simple guide on how to change your diet and a lot of important information about the subject of Sorbitol.

Read about fascinating background information, scientific findings, experience reports and secret tips which are tailor-made for you relating to your Sorbitol intolerance and which are designed to help you to achieve a healthy, longer and more fulfilling life.

This book is available on Amazon!

DISCLAIMER

©2019, Lutz Schneider

1st Edition

All rights reserved. Reprinting, of all or part of this book, is not permitted. No part of this book may be reproduced or copied in any form or by any means without written permission from the author or publisher. Publisher: GbR, Martin Seidel und Corinna Krupp, Bachstraße 37, 53498 Bad Breisig, Germany, email: info@expertengruppeverlag.de, Cover photo: www.depositphoto.com. The information provided within this book is for general information purposes only. It does not represent any recommendation or application of the methods mentioned within. The information in this book does not purport to imply or guarantee its completeness, accuracy, or topicality. This book in no way replaces the competent recommendations of, or care given by, a doctor. The author and publisher do not assume and hereby disclaims any liability for damages or disruption caused by the use of the information given herein